LOWERING
HIGH BLOOD
PRESSURE

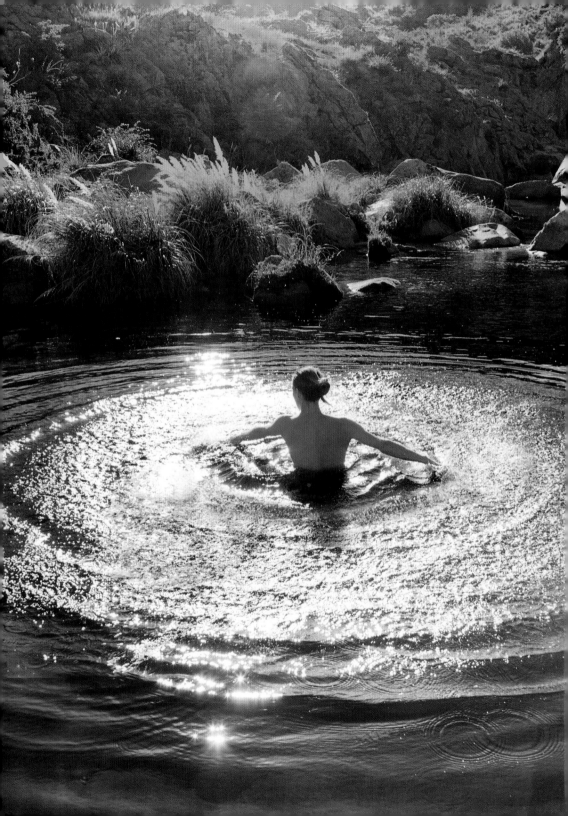

LOWERING HIGH BLOOD PRESSURE

The Three-type Holistic Approach

Dr Thomas Breitkreuz & Annette Bopp

Floris Books

Translated by Catherine Creegar

First published in German as *Bluthochdruck Senken:
Das 3-Typen-Konzept* in 2009 by Gräfe und Unzer Verlag

Translated from the first edition and published in English
by Floris Books in 2014
© 2009 Gräfe und Unzer Verlag, GmbH, Munich
Translation © Floris Books 2014, Edinburgh 2014

 Also available as an eBook

British Library CIP Data available
ISBN 978-178250-119-0
Printed in China through Asia Pacific Offset Ltd

Contents

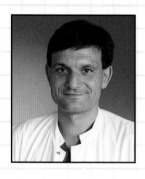

DR THOMAS BREITKREUZ

Dr Thomas Breitkreuz was Chief Physician in the department of internal medicine at Herdecke Community Hospital, Germany, from 2001 to 2010. Since then he has been Chief Physician at Paracelsus Hospital, Germany. He specialises in anthroposophical medical treatments for high blood pressure and cancer.

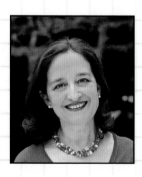

ANNETTE BOPP

Annette Bopp trained as a biologist and is now a freelance medical journalist. Her writing has been widely published in Germany and she leads the editorial board of medical magazine *Medizin Individuell*.

'Lifestyle is more important than medication, and actions you take yourself are often more important than prescriptions.'

Foreword

High blood pressure (hypertension) is one of the most common chronic illnesses in the world and one of the chief causes of cardiovascular disease, which in turn is one of the most frequent causes of death – reason enough to tackle your high blood pressure.

In recent years, our understanding of how to treat high blood pressure has fundamentally changed. Steps patients can take on their own have become more important than medical treatment, and lifestyle changes more important than prescriptions. This new understanding, combined with many years of treating and talking to patients, led to an updated treatment model: the three-type approach to high blood pressure. This individualised approach, which is now being implemented in many medical practices and anthroposophical clinics, incorporates options derived from naturopathy, anthroposophical medicine, and conventional medicine.

What's more, this programme is fun! Instead of attempting to reduce the statistical risk of cardiovascular disease, it aims to change your life right here and now, by balancing out any one-sided aspects of your individual constitution. The result is lower blood pressure and fundamental improvements in your quality of life. We're talking about concrete, individualised steps you can take, and you are the centre of this therapeutic approach. It works fast, so you will soon enjoy increased productivity and resilience. In particular, you'll find that you're simply enjoying life more – much more. Just try it!

Dr Thomas Breitkreuz
Annette Bopp

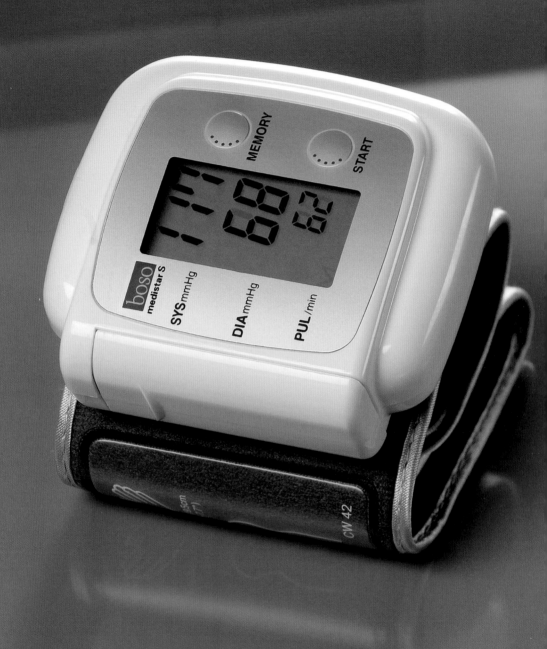

PART ONE

Theory

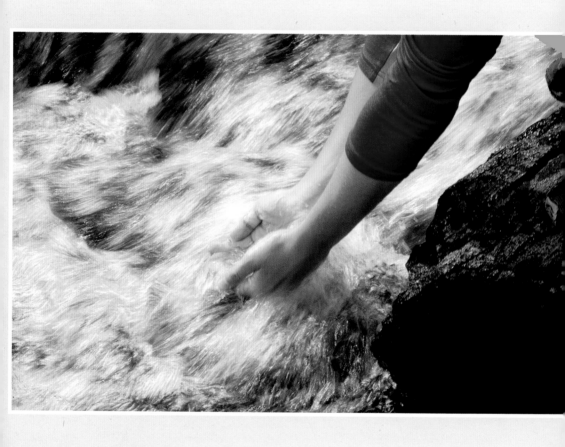

Blood Pressure and Health

Why our blood is pressurised

Anything that flows must be pressurised or it would not be able to move, so our blood needs pressure in order to circulate throughout the body. We need blood pressure in order to stand upright, to move, to think – in short, to *live*. Without pressure, blood could not to rise into the head against the force of gravity. That's why we lose consciousness if our blood pressure drops steeply. Adequate blood pressure, therefore, is essential for an active life.

Blood pressure varies constantly

Our blood pressure is constantly changing, resetting itself with every heartbeat as our bodies adapt to the circumstances of our lives. Blood pressure is lower when we are sleeping than when we are awake. To allow us to wake up, the body raises our blood pressure an hour or two before waking. Sympathetic nervous system activity increases, and as a result the heart beats faster and the tension in the vascular muscles increases. At this stage, even our dreams reveal that we are beginning to 'come to' – the closer we are to waking up, the more realistic our dreams become. In contrast, dreams during the first few hours of sleep are more imaginative and less lifelike.

Blood pressure is lower when we are lying down than when we are sitting or standing. When we stand up, however, an abrupt increase in blood pressure is required in order to keep the brain adequately supplied. In some individuals, this increase doesn't happen rapidly enough, and they tend to 'see black' briefly when they stand up.

When we move and tense our muscles, the blood supply to the muscles must increase, which also requires an increase in blood pressure – enough to ensure even tensed muscles remain well supplied.

After a meal, blood supply to the gastrointestinal tract increases by a factor of three to four, and maintaining the usual level of blood pressure in the brain takes more effort, which is why we may feel like resting after we eat. The less fluid there is circulating throughout the body, the lower our blood pressure drops and the more the tension increases in the small arteries, which are forced to contract in order to maintain blood pressure in spite of the reduced volume of blood. The heart has to beat faster in order to keep this smaller amount of blood in circulation. In extreme cases, circulation may fail altogether because adequate blood pressure can no longer be maintained, and the person loses consciousness. That is why adequate fluid intake is important every day.

When the kidneys excrete increased amounts of salt and fluid, blood pressure drops. Conversely, the kidneys can also raise blood pressure by retaining salt and fluid. They do this by secreting a protein called renin. Renin is an enzyme that contributes to the formation of angiotensin, a hormone that constricts the blood vessels and stimulates the adrenal glands to release another hormone called aldosterone. Aldosterone causes the kidneys to eliminate less salt, meaning more salt is retained in the

Blood pressure and consciousness

Adequate blood pressure allows us to maintain consciousness. Conversely, we lose consciousness when the pressure drops excessively. An example is when teenagers faint at rock concerts out of sheer enthusiasm: they 'lose consciousness' – i.e., consciousness no longer resides in the body. When this happens, the blood vessels dilate, especially in peripheral parts of the body. Blood pressure drops, and blood supply to the brain is no longer adequate. A few seconds in a horizontal position with legs raised is all it takes to restore consciousness.

body and blood pressure rises as a result. Blocking this mechanism causes blood pressure to drop. This principle underlies the action of many blood pressure medications (see pages 143–157).

Psychological influences and stress also influence blood pressure by affecting the tension in the blood vessels, which dilate or contract in response. This is as true of happiness and pleasure as it is of worry, anger, and sorrow. Blood pressure rises with every extreme emotion and drops again as soon as the tension passes or an escape hatch is found.

Blood pressure adjusts with every heartbeat, constantly oscillating around a specific base value. This variability of blood pressure, which allows it to adapt to every situation, is an important for stable circulation.

Circulation and blood vessels

Blood circulates constantly through the vessels, with the heart in the centre of the system. In terms of function, the circulatory system as a whole is divided into three parts: head circulation, lung circulation, and limb circulation.

Relatively speaking, head circulation is more autonomous than the other two branches of the system. The brain is capable of maintaining constant pressure in the blood vessels that supply its neurons, which ensures both an adequate supply of blood and constant consciousness. As with all brain-regulated functions, whether we are resting, running, or excited makes no difference. The influence of bodily processes on conscious thinking, feeling, and willing is deliberately minimised, and this emancipation contributes to our autonomy as human beings. Maintaining a consistent blood pressure, to the extent possible, is also important for the brain's supply of oxygen. The brain alone consumes a quarter of the blood's oxygen content! At high blood pressure levels over 230–240 mmHg for the systolic (upper) reading and 130 mmHg for the diastolic (lower), relatively constant blood pressure can no longer be maintained in the head (see page 24). Typical symptoms of a 'hypertensive crisis' of this sort are headache, nausea, dizziness, and even paralysis or coordination disturbances. If blood pressure continues to rise, convulsions may occur. All of these symptoms are expressions of the fact that brain function has been affected, which is why they are similar to the symptoms of stroke.

The structure of arteries and veins

There are two distinctly different types of blood vessel: arteries, which lead away from the heart, and veins, which lead back towards the heart. Arteries transport primarily oxygen-rich blood that exits the left ventricle via the aorta to enter the head and body. Only the pulmonary artery transports oxygen-poor blood from the right ventricle to the lungs, where it releases carbon dioxide in the pulmonary alveoli and absorbs oxygen before flowing back to the heart (left ventricle) via the pulmonary vein and then on to the head and body.

At 40 cm (16 in) in length and 2–2.5 cm (1 in) in diameter, the aorta is the body's largest blood vessel. It originates in the left ventricle and divides into ever-finer branches and twigs throughout the body.

Three circulatory systems

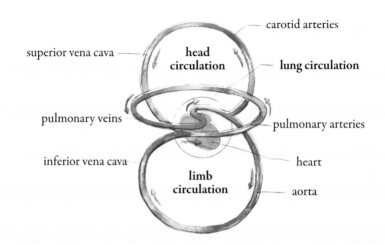

The circulatory system as a whole consists of head circulation, pulmonary circulation, and limb circulation.

Arteries

Arteries are made up of three layers: the inner vascular wall (intima) is a very thin, sensitive membrane with an extremely smooth surface that presents minimal resistance to the free flow of blood. The middle layer (media) consists of soft, smooth muscle cells and a network of elastic fibres. These muscles are not subject to voluntary control; they contract and relax in response to impulses from the nervous system or to changes in temperature. A fibrous outer layer of connective tissue (adventitia) connects each artery to the surrounding tissue and is criss-crossed by a network of nerves that conduct the impulses, triggering contraction or relaxation of the muscle cells.

Veins are made up of two layers. Their walls are thinner than those of arteries and consist of a very thin internal membrane and a surrounding layer of muscle. Many veins, especially in the legs, are equipped with valves that intersect the length at specific intervals. These valves ensure that the blood can flow in only one direction, towards the heart, rather than back down into the legs or arms. Veins look bluish and are readily visible on the temples and on the backs of the hands and feet, since they are often located just below the skin. Arteries are used for palpating the pulse and checking blood pressure, but blood samples are drawn from veins, because the blood would actively gush out of arteries.

Blood vessels: a finely branching network

Arteries and veins run throughout the body like a fine mesh net. The combined length of all the blood vessels totals 140,000 km (87,000 miles), which is roughly three and a half times the Earth's circumference. Their total surface area is 6,000–7,000 square metres (65,000–75,350 square feet) – about the size of a football pitch! There are 40 major arteries with 600 branches, which continue branching to form 1,800 small arteries, 40 million arterioles, and 1.2 billion capillaries, each with a length of 0.5 to 4 mm (½–2 in). The venous network is similarly complex, with approximately 80 million venules merging into 1800 vein 'twigs', 600 vein branches, and finally into the 40 major veins that empty into the venae cavae.

Capillaries

Capillaries are the tiny, delicate terminal vessels in the arterial system; they form the connections between arteries and veins. Capillaries are made up of only two layers, a thin inner membrane and a surrounding layer of protective cells. Due to its very fine branching, the capillary zone accounts for almost 60% of the total surface area of the blood vessels. Blood pressure in the capillaries is minimal and barely measurable. This is where tissues are nourished, as if by well-drained forest soil. Since blood pressure here is too low to move the fluid, it seeps out of the capillaries into the surrounding tissue and is then reabsorbed into the capillaries. The amount of fluid involved and its components depend on concentrations present in the surroundings. This is where oxygen is released and carbon dioxide is taken up; fats are bound to proteins to form lipoproteins; minerals and trace elements are exchanged in a constant give-and-take of substances. All growth and regeneration takes place in this zone of barely measurable blood pressure. Getting the blood to this point, however, depends on pressure and the pulsing action of the heart.

Veins

Blood from the capillary zone is then absorbed into the venules to be transported back to the heart through the venous system. The venous system is pressurised by suction that results from breathing: when the lungs and ribcage expand, negative pressure allows the blood to flow upwards. Veins are also subjected to pressure from the movements of the skeletal muscles that surround them and from the pulsation of adjacent arteries (two veins

Did you know...

...that the distended bellies of malnourished people are the result of protein deficiency? When protein is lacking, fluids cannot be reabsorbed from the capillaries into the bloodstream. In contrast, the legs and arms become mere skin and bones due to muscle loss, which is also due to protein deficiency.

run alongside each artery). That's why physical activity is so important for good 'venous return' of blood from the arms and legs back to the heart.

How blood pressure comes about

Blood pressure is the pressure that moves the blood through the arteries. Blood always flows from areas of higher pressure to areas of lower pressure. This is a basic law of physics that also applies to weather. For example, in meteorology a low pressure area pulls air in from a high pressure area. In the arteries, pressure is determined by the amount of blood, the beating of the heart, and the resistance the flow of blood encounters in the vessels. Resistance in the tiny arterioles far away from the heart is a crucial factor: when they are not elastic enough to contract, blood pressure cannot develop effectively. Right down into their smallest branches, the arteries need a certain amount of tension to allow the blood to flow into their terminal branches.

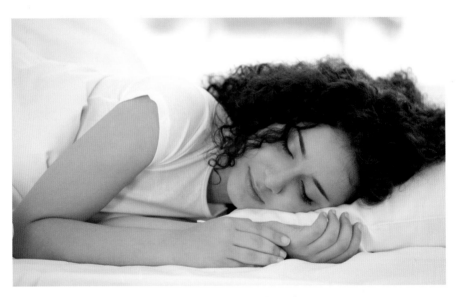

Blood pressure drops after lunch – an ideal time to lie down for a nap!

The blood pressure waltz

Blood pressure is subject to a specific daily rhythm, rising and falling as if in a waltz. It drops to its lowest point around 3 am, the 'biological midnight' when sleep is deepest. Beginning around 4 am, our blood pressure begins to rise, first slowly (to prepare us for waking up) and then abruptly (when the alarm goes off) so we are then able to stand up. Because our blood pressure remains relatively high throughout the morning, that's when we are normally most productive. Blood pressure drops after lunch, so we tend to feel tired then, and a brief nap makes good sense. After that, blood pressure rises again, reaching its second peak around 7 pm before dropping again.

Nocturnal blood pressure

At night, a significant drop (or 'dip') in blood pressure is normal and a sign that the body has entered an effective restorative phase. Night-time blood pressure readings should be at least 10% lower (but less than 20% lower) than the daytime average ('normal dipper'). Fluctuations of less than 10% ('non-dipper') or over 20% ('extreme dipper') are associated with an increased danger of organ damage in hypertensive patients. In other words, both are indications of risk, as is blood pressure that is higher at night than during the day ('inverted dipper').

It's all in the rhythm

Blood pressure that can fluctuate effectively is an indicator of circulatory stability. Women have the advantage here: their blood pressure is more adaptable, due to their monthly cycle. Elasticity begins to decline only after menopause, which is why many women experience an increase in blood pressure then. This tendency, however, is easy to counteract with a rhythmical daily routine, as proved by a study of Italian nuns. Physicians monitored the blood pressure of 144 Benedictine nuns and a control group of 138 women from the general population over a period of 20 years. In the control group, average blood pressure rose from 130/80 mmHg at the beginning of the study to 165/100 at the end, but in the group of Benedictines it remained at 130/80 and none of the nuns developed high blood pressure. Factors such as familial high blood pressure, cardiovascular disease, weight, and consumption of salt, tea, and coffee were comparable, as were pre or post-menopausal status and educational levels. In other words, there were no significant differences between the two groups.

The only explanation for the observed difference in blood pressure is that the nuns were living an isolated life in absolute stillness in their idyllic, cloistered location. The course of their days, weeks, months, and years was rhythmically structured and had been shaped for hundreds of years by the alternation of prayer and work ('ora et labora') at consistent, predetermined times. Nuns also do not question the meaning of their life; they are firmly anchored in their order, living their faith.

In contrast to nuns, ordinary women are exposed to many stressors. They have careers and households to attend to, and many have partners and children as well. Concerns about work, stress within the family, financial needs, noise, pollution, and other environmental influences accompany them every day. Although the recurrence of annual holidays such as Easter and Christmas and the change of seasons do provide some rhythm to their years, their daily routine is much more unstructured than that of nuns. It would be unrealistic to suggest that we all ought to model our schedules on life in a cloister, but we can still take this highly structured life as an ideal or example. You can learn more starting on page 129.

The daily routine in a cloister

In a Benedictine cloister, the day is rhythmically subdivided. Practical activity and spiritual reflection alternate repeatedly, as the example below shows.

5:45 a.m.	Get up
6:00 a.m.	First prayer of the day (Prime)
6:30 a.m.	Assembly, continuation of prayers, work assignments, breakfast
8:00 a.m.	Work in various areas
9:00 a.m.	Prayer of the third hour of the day (Terce)
9:00 a.m.	Mass, followed by work
11:30 a.m.	Prayer of the sixth hour of the day (Sext)
12:00 noon	Lunch and rest period
2:00 p.m.	Prayer of the ninth hour of the day (None)
2:30 p.m.	Work
4:30 p.m.	Evensong (Vespers)
5:30 p.m.	Evening meal; sharing of the day's events
7:30 p.m.	Spiritual reading
8:00 p.m.	Compline (prayer), followed by lights-out

The right way to check blood pressure

If your doctor is checking your blood pressure for the first time, make sure he or she does it on both arms. If there is a difference of more than 5 mmHg, the higher pressure is the one that counts. Sometimes the presence of a narrow section of artery somewhere above the cuff (in the chest, near the collarbone, or in the upper arm) can lower the pressure and throw the reading off.

How blood pressure is measured

Blood pressure is typically measured using an inflatable cuff on the upper arm. Attached to this is a rubber ball that serves as a bellows, which is used to inflate the cuff until the artery in the arm is pressed completely closed. This can be somewhat uncomfortable – the higher the pressure, the stronger the pinching sensation in the arm becomes. This pressure registers on a manometer connected to the bellows. At the same time, the health care practitioner places the membrane of a stethoscope on the inside of the elbow to listen for the pulse beat. No pulse can be heard when the artery is completely closed.

Then air is released from the cuff to unblock the artery. The more slowly this is done, the more accurate the reading will be. As soon as the blood begins flowing again, the sound of the pulse can be heard. The pulse corresponds to the heartbeat, developing when the left ventricle contracts (systole) and propels blood into the aorta. The pressure at the instant when the first pulse is heard is the top – systolic – number in a blood pressure reading. The air continues to be let out of the cuff slowly until the sound of the pulse subsides completely. This is the moment when the left ventricle expands to receive blood from the atrium (diastole). This pressure is recorded as the bottom – diastolic – number in a blood pressure reading.

So the pressure reading on the manometer corresponds to the pressure in the artery. It is recorded in millimeters of mercury (mmHg for short), the height of the column of mercury that would produce it. In other words, 1mmHg is the pressure produced by a column of mercury one millimeter in height.

Check it yourself – properly!

Checking your blood pressure at home has become common, and it makes sense to keep track. The most commonly available devices check blood pressure at the wrist. Make sure the brand has been tested for accuracy before you buy. Other than that, there are just a few important tips to ensure accurate readings:

☞　Sit quietly for five or ten minutes before checking your blood pressure. If you check right after physical activity (climbing stairs, for example), the reading will be high.

☞　Take your blood pressure sitting down, and use the same arm your doctor selected as giving the correct reading (see box opposite).

☞　Make sure the cuff fits snugly and hold your arm still while the machine is running.

☞　Hold your arm at heart height (not lower and not higher) while measuring, or the device will not yield a correct reading.

☞　If you want to redo the test, wait 30 seconds to a minute before repeating the procedure.

If you have a blood pressure meter with an upper arm cuff, place the cuff approximately two finger-widths above the crook of your arm and leave enough space to insert two fingers under the cuff – that way the inflation will create enough pressure but won't be too painful. It's best to sit at a table, place the blood pressure meter on it and rest your forearm

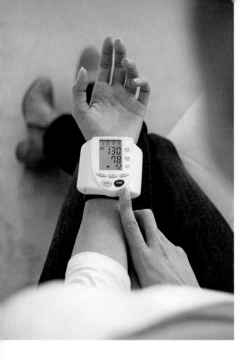

on the table, which will naturally put the lower edge of the cuff at the right level (heart height). The cuff needs to be the right size for the circumference of your upper arm; an extra-large size is available if needed.

Be sure to follow proper procedures for checking your blood pressure.

Normal and elevated blood pressure readings at rest

	Upper figure in mmHG	Lower figure in mmHg
Optimum blood pressure	120	80
Normal blood pressure	< 130	< 85
Still normal	130–139	85–89
Isolated elevated systolic blood pressure	> 140	< 90
Borderline elevated blood pressure	140–149	90–94
Mildly elevated blood pressure	150–159	90–99
Moderately elevated blood pressure	160–179	100–109
Severely elevated blood pressure	> 180	> 110
Hypertensive crisis (life-threatening)	> 230	> 130

What drives blood pressure up?

In certain situations, blood pressure *has* to go up so the body can meet the demands being placed on it. Examples include:

☞ Racing to catch a bus or train that's about to pull away.

☞ Dangerous traffic situations that require quick reactions.

☞ Any situation requiring a high level of alertness and concentration. The situation can be positive: the high blood pressure that accompanies initial stage fright 'sets the stage' for a good performance.

☞ Threatening events that necessitate sudden flight.

☞ During sex. Blood pressure tends to rise more in men than in women, and affectionate, pleasurable love-making drives blood pressure up less rapidly than libidinous, primarily climax-oriented sex.

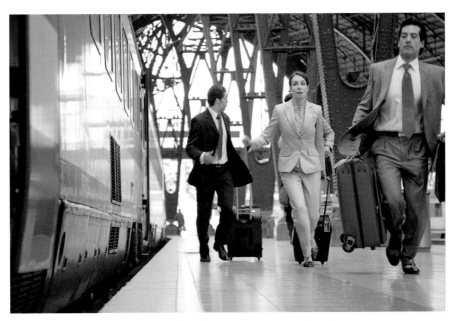

Hurrying to catch the train causes a brief but significant rise in blood pressure.

25

Stress drives blood pressure up

When we're in a rush, even red traffic lights cause blood pressure to increase. That's why couriers and truck drivers, with their consistently tight schedules of pick-ups and deliveries, are especially likely to have high blood pressure. For them every red light is a significant source of stress. Anyone exposed to this type of stress for eight hours a day or longer is working under tremendous pressure.

This means it is essential for our blood pressure to be able to rise sharply for brief periods of time, since that's the only way we can be ready for action at any moment. This is a capability granted primarily to humans; it is less evident in animals. Our need for an elevated level of basic tension in order to be able to take action at any moment has to do with the fact that we guide our activity willfully and deliberately, not instinctively and reflexively, as animals do. Only our blood pressure can ensure our full presence as spirit, soul, and body, with the associated degree of readiness for action. For example, a hunter lying in wait in a raised blind, ready to ambush a big buck, is under constant pressure. His spiking blood pressure and rapidly beating heart ensure that he will be able to respond and shoot the second the animal emerges from the underbrush.

Building up suspense

Being engrossed in a gripping movie or TV show or on the verge of identifying the murderer in a mystery novel can also raise blood pressure.

But if this phase persists for hours, it increases the risk that the body will no longer be able to withstand the stress. Death could suddenly overtake that hunter, if persistent high blood pressure triggers a heart attack or stroke.

Being on heightened alert for long periods of time is not healthy. Stress that persists for weeks, months, or even years is a very significant risk factor for cardiovascular disease.

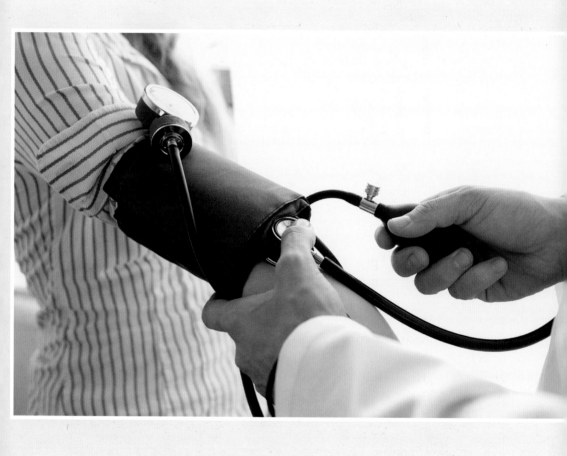

The Consequences of High Blood Pressure

Persistent high blood pressure is a sign of the body's struggle to maintain its autonomy as it encounters obstacles that limit the blood pressure's normal variability. Examples of such obstacles are: a constant flood of stimuli that places excessive demands on our senses and makes us nervous and fidgety; an excess of foods that overload the digestive tract; years of stress at home or at work, which leads to a feeling of helplessness. Constantly suppressing anger and aggression leads to persistent tension.

Initially, high blood pressure is actually a healthy response. The body resorts to higher blood pressure in an attempt to overcome opposition and preserve its independence. If the condition persists for a long time, however, it takes on a life of its own and becomes chronic. The body 'forgets' that there is any other way to live. Ultimately, therefore, high blood pressure becomes a disease with potentially life-threatening consequences.

Lack of exercise, obesity, diabetes, smoking, and genetic predisposition can also drive blood pressure up. In many cases, combinations of mutually reinforcing factors are involved. For example, people often attempt to compensate for stress by overeating and then gain weight.

High blood pressure is neither a purely bodily problem nor an unavoidable fate. It's more a question of culture. It's important to ask yourself: under existing circumstances, how can I organise my life in a way that supports me both psychologically and physically? How can I balance out my weaknesses and one-sided tendencies and apply my strengths in ways that help me rather than harm me? Medication is not the only treatment option – it is just one among many.

A stealthy process

In people under 50, high blood pressure often begins with elevated diastolic readings – that is, the lower number is above 90 mmHg – which is an expression of increased tension in the arterioles, especially when the rise in blood pressure is due to persistent stress. As a result of narrowing of the blood vessels, these individuals usually have the pale skin typical of stress types (see page 48). Alternatively, high blood pressure can be accompanied by a pronounced abundance of blood, as shown by a florid complexion, purplish ears, haemorrhoids, bulging veins in the legs, and sensitivity to cold. This 'red' high blood pressure is typical of the abdominal type (see page 52).

High systolic readings (over 140mmHg) appear primarily during acute stress, whether physical (such as while bicycling uphill or mountain climbing) or psychological (such as during arguments or unpleasant conversations).

Check it several times

If your blood pressure is abnormally high when you check it, repeat the test several times at intervals of at least two minutes. Make sure you are sitting quietly. If all the readings taken then and later in the day are too high, consult your doctor.

Many people are remain unaware that their high blood pressure is high because for a long time it causes either no symptoms or only symptoms that one would not usually associate with high blood pressure (such as morning headaches and dizziness). People with strong self-awareness may also notice a strange 'whirring' sensation in the head and an inexplicable increase in irritability or inner restlessness.

Blood vessel damage

Persistent elevated blood pressure damages arteries in two ways. First, sites where the delicate inner membrane is torn become locations for deposition of plaque; second, persistent tension in the muscle walls causes the arteries to lose elasticity.

Especially in the early stages, deposits on the artery walls are covered by a thin, easily damaged membrane. If this membrane ruptures, the contents spill out and exert an almost magnetic attraction on blood platelets (thrombocytes), which combine with the components of plaque to form a blood clot. This obstacle traps other components of the blood, so the plug increases rapidly in size until it either completely blocks the blood vessel or breaks loose and is carried along by the blood stream until it lodges in some smaller blood vessel. Heart attacks are caused by clots

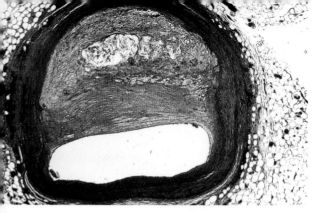

blocking coronary arteries, which are responsible for the blood supply to the heart muscle. Clots that form in the carotid arteries or arteries in the brain produce strokes.

Cross-section of an artery greatly narrowed by deposits.

Organ damage

Damage to blood vessels caused by high blood pressure not only increases the risk of heart attack and stroke, but can also cause damage to the heart, brain, kidneys, and eyes. The most important secondary disorders are:

☞ Cardiac insufficiency: the extra effort of years of pumping against considerable circulatory resistance due to high blood pressure increases the muscle mass of the left ventricle. Even before an ultrasound can reveal thickening of the cardiac wall, the heart can be losing elasticity. In particular, it is no longer capable of expanding to its fullest, and its passive phase – when there is no resistance to the inflowing blood – is disrupted. As a result, the ventricle takes in less blood and ejects less into the blood stream. The heart must then beat faster to maintain circulation. Over time, a vicious cycle develops and the heart becomes progressively weaker.

☞ Cardiac arrhythmias: cardiac insufficiency often leads to a specific form of cardiac arrhythmia called *atrial fibrillation*. When the ventricle resists filling completely, the atrium pumps harder in response and becomes exhausted and dilated, which disrupts the network of muscle fibres that conduct the electrical impulses that trigger heartbeats. As a result, these impulses are no longer evenly distributed but occur in chaotic bursts that make the atrium 'fibrillate', contracting 500 or more times per minute, then almost stopping. As a result, the filling of the ventricle becomes even more uneven. But an already weakened heart depends on the atrium functioning well, or the ventricle's fill level will be reduced even more. Atrial fibrillation can reduce cardiac output by an additional 20%. It also increases the risk of stroke due to the tendency of clots to form in no-flow zones in the lobes of the atrium. These clots then break loose and are carried away by the blood stream. They usually end up in the brain, because the blood expelled from the left ventricle goes straight from the aorta into the arteries that supply the head.

☞ Cerebral hemorrhage: cerebral hemorrhage, or hemorrhagic stroke, is another form of stroke due to rupturing of fragile arteries in the brain. (The other form occurs when a clot blocks a brain artery, cutting off the oxygen supply to adjacent areas.)

☞ Dementia: brain deficiencies in the form of dementia can be due to decreased blood supply that results from arteriosclerosis. The signs of it are conspicuous forgetfulness and significantly compromised concentration associated with disorientation.

☞ Kidney failure: when the kidneys are poorly supplied with blood, they can no longer serve their filtration function effectively and secrete too much protein. Initially, the protein loss is relatively minor (microalbuminuria), but later it increases (proteinuria) and leads to significantly reduced kidney function: up to and including kidney failure.

☞ Changes in the retina, vision disturbances: in the long term, narrowing of arteries in the retina of the eye leads to vision disturbances or even to permanent, irreparable retinal damage.

Atrial fibrillation

If you notice your heart repeatedly skipping beats and beating very irregularly for extended periods, you should ask your primary care physician for a referral to a cardiologist. These symptoms could be due to atrial fibrillation, which results from cardiac insufficiency and high blood pressure and must be treated.

What women should know

Up to age 35, only 1½–2% of women have high blood pressure, but after menopause the percentage increases to more than 40%. Two-thirds of all women between the ages of 30 and 50 do not know their blood pressure, but there are several important factors that women in this particular age group need to consider.

☞ The synthetic hormones in the contraceptive pill drive blood pressure up in one in three women under age 35, especially if they smoke (which means oral contraceptives should actually be off-limits to smokers) and all the more so when their parents or siblings already have (or had) high blood pressure. That's why blood pressure should be monitored repeatedly during the first few months of taking the pill, even if it has always been normal or on the low side.

☞ 5–10% of all pregnant women experience severe increases in blood pressure during the last trimester of pregnancy (pre-eclampsia, formerly also known as toxemia of pregnancy). In these cases, there is a danger that the baby will no longer be adequately supplied with nutrients and oxygen via the placenta and will have to be delivered prematurely by caesarean section. For this reason, pregnant women need to monitor their blood pressure especially frequently and their physicians should use diagnostic test strips to check for protein in the urine (microalbuminuria) in order to identify gestational hypertension as early as possible.

☞ Blood pressure rises in many women during menopause as estrogen levels drop. Until menopause, this hormonal 'vascular protection' is needed because the blood vessels need to be able to adapt to the increase in circulating blood volume – one and a half times the usual amount

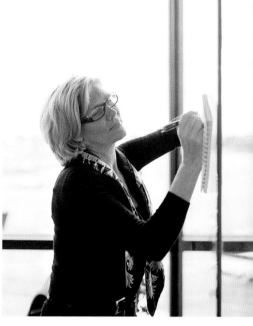

Women should pay special attention to their blood pressure during and after menopause.

– that occurs during pregnancy. After menopause, this protective mechanism is no longer necessary and the arteries sacrifice some of their resilience.

☞ During and after menopause, therefore, it is important to monitor your blood pressure repeatedly, even if your blood pressure was formerly on the low side.

Primary and secondary high blood pressure

In roughly 90% of cases, there is no organic cause of high blood pressure; it develops as a result of external influences and constitutional traits (primary hypertension). In 5–15% of hypertensive patients, high blood pressure is a consequence of another illness (secondary hypertension).

☞ When the renal artery narrows by more than 40%, the kidney is no longer well supplied with blood, and in response, it activates the hormones renin and angiotensin, which induce a rise in blood pressure in the arterioles and increased retention of fluid in the kidney. As a result, the volume of blood increases and blood supply improves, not only in the kidneys but throughout the body. 'Renal artery stenosis' of this type is found in approximately one in every hundred hypertensive patients. In women under 55, it is usually caused by fibromuscular dysplasia (thickening of the connective tissue in the renal arteries).

☞ Kidney disorders such as cysts, fibrosis, cancer, or chronic inflammation can have consequences similar to those of renal artery stenosis.

☞ One in every five cases of hyperthyroidism leads to systolic hypertension (see page 24), while hypothyroidism can increase diastolic pressure.

☞ Very high blood pressure readings of 170/120 mmHg that do not respond to the usual medications (ACE inhibitors and angiotensin receptor blockers) are typical of Conn's syndrome, in which the adrenals produce excessive amounts of the hormone aldosterone. Other hormonal imbalances that result in high blood pressure include tumors of the adrenal cortex (pheochromocytoma) and increased secretion of cortisone in functional disorders of the adrenal cortex (Cushing syndrome). 24-hour urine tests for concentrations of these hormones are used to identify such diseases.

☞ Malformations of the aorta can also lead to high blood pressure.

☞ All of these possibilities should be ruled out by your doctor before a diagnosis of primary hypertension can be made.

Prompt treatment

The longer high blood pressure remains untreated, the greater the possible damage. For example, high blood pressure precedes 50% of fatal heart attacks and 90% of strokes. That's why it's important to maintain healthy blood pressure levels. There's more to it than just the numbers, however. Your blood pressure's natural variability is even more important.

24-hour blood pressure monitoring

To diagnose high blood pressure effectively, your doctor can arrange for 24-hour blood pressure monitoring. It's done with the usual upper arm cuff, which inflates every fifteen minutes (every 30 minutes at night) and sends the data to a small recording device. In addition, you keep a diary about the day's activities and events. The data is evaluated once the monitoring is complete. The average of all readings should be no higher than 135/86 mmHg, there should be a significant difference between day and night readings, and your blood pressure should be able to adapt to different situations during the day.

What your doctor should check

When chronic high blood pressure is suspected, the following tests and examinations are essential. Your doctor should:

☞ Ask you about your medical history, your current lifestyle, and any problems that are weighing on you.

☞ Give you a complete physical examination: listen to your heart and certain blood vessels with the stethoscope and take your pulse with his/her fingers. Of course that process can be automated, but a doctor's fingers can also sense pulse quality and draw conclusions about cardiac function.

☞ Check your blood pressure in both arms and arrange for 24-hour monitoring (see previous page). A fifth of all blood pressure readings taken in doctors' offices are false highs ('white coat' syndrome, due to nervousness) while one quarter are too low (due to the doctor's calming influence), so 24-hour monitoring is essential to an accurate diagnosis.

☞ Order ultrasounds of your heart and kidneys. The ultrasound image of your heart (echocardiogram) reveals any thickening of the heart muscle due to high blood pressure. In addition, the doctor can tell whether the heart valves are closing properly and whether there are any signs of poor blood supply to the heart muscle.

☞ Order blood tests for: creatinine (kidney function), lipid profile (total cholesterol, HDL, LDL, triglycerides), thyroid hormone, renin, aldosterone, sodium, potassium.

☞ Order an eye exam. The ophthalmologist must check whether the fundus of the eye is still well supplied with blood. The fundus is the only place in the body where any narrowing of the small arteries can be observed directly.

The condition of these arteries allows conclusions to be drawn about the situation in the brain.

☞ Test your urine for sugar and protein. A glucose tolerance test is in order if diabetes is suspected or a genetic predisposition exists.

☞ Additional tests may be required, such as hormone tests or ultrasounds of the kidney arteries.

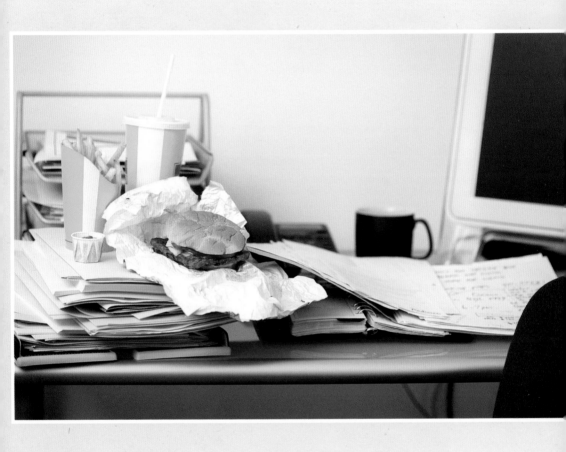

Lifestyle and Blood Pressure

Our modern western lifestyle favours the development of high blood pressure. Five factors in particular have been implicated. They can all have an adverse effect on blood pressure.

Lack of physical activity

In the past hundred years, human life has undergone radical changes. Thanks to cars, trains and aeroplanes, we now cover great distances with breathtaking speed, without moving ourselves. Escalators and elevators have replaced stairs in our urban buildings. We drive or take public transport to work or to go shopping. Even in agriculture, most of the work is now done by machines. This lack of physical exertion has enormous advantages, because the wear and tear on our joints and spines is greatly reduced. On the other hand, though, we are becoming more inactive, which has effects on the body as a whole and promotes obesity, especially as food is now more abundant and calorie-rich than ever before.

Obesity

In terms of the variety and richness of our food, we have never had it so good. In combination with lack of movement, however, this abundance results in deposits of fat, especially in the abdominal cavity, because the body simply doesn't use up all the energy it gets from food. Normally, fat is deposited in fatty tissues just under the skin, where it serves as a warmth-conserving layer. This type of padding is not dangerous, nor are round buttocks or broad hips in women. But fat cells (adipocytes) are only deposited in the abdominal

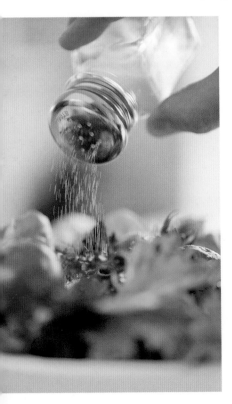

cavity in cases of excess, when too much food (or alcohol) is available. Then the body makes too many triglycerides, and its only way of coping with them is to deposit them in fat cells; in this case, in the abdominal cavity. Abdominal fat is highly active. It activates blood clotting and generates increased amounts of substances that enhance growth or attract inflammatory cells. All fat cells have the potential do this, but in this respect abdominal fat is four times as active as other adipose tissues. Increased inflammation and activated blood clotting, however, are the stuff of arteriosclerosis – hardening of the arteries – and of deposits and blood clots that block the arteries, which are the primary cause of heart attacks and strokes. That's why excess abdominal fat is one of the most important risk factors for cardiovascular disease.

Go easy on the salt – it can drive up your blood pressure.

Check your waist measurement

Your waist measurement is an indicator of your risk of developing cardiovascular disease. Take this measurement halfway between the top of your hip bone and the lower edge of your ribs, i.e., just above the navel. Stand up straight and exhale before measuring. For a woman, the measuring tape should show not more than 88 cm (35 in); for a man, not more than 102 cm (40 in). These numbers, however, are higher in about 50% of the population. When no other risk factors are present, a few extra centimetres or inches are not cause for concern.

Melt away abdominal fat

The best way to melt away abdominal fat is to exercise to the point of sweating at least once a day. It makes no difference whether you exercise in the morning, at noon, or in the evening, and it doesn't matter whether you climb stairs or go jogging through the park. Fat is burned only through active movement that creates plenty of heat. Fasting also melts away cushions of fat, but fat lost during fasting typically returns rather quickly.

Stress and smoking

The sympathetic nervous system enhances attentiveness and motivation, and severe stress makes it function at full throttle. The result is a persistent increase in tension in the small arteries far away from the heart, which constrict, increasing resistance. Blood pressure rises, especially the lower (diastolic) number. The greater the basic tension, however, the less capable of variation your blood becomes, because it is in a constant state of upregulation. Increased tension in the sympathetic nervous system also causes secretion of the hormone angiotensin, which narrows small blood vessels in particular, raising blood pressure even more.

The constituents of tobacco smoke also contribute to high blood pressure by damaging the internal membranes of arteries, which promotes arteriosclerosis (see page 31).

Is it really just genetic?

In 2008, newspapers reported that scientists in the US had discovered that the STK39 gene was responsible for susceptibility to high blood pressure. At the time of this book's publication, the article was available to read online at http://www.pnas.org/content/106/1/226.abstract. The researchers estimate that one in five Europeans carries this gene variant. In fact, a genetic component does play a role in many cases of high blood pressure, but it's a risk factor, not a cause: no one is at the mercy of his or her genes. If you have close relatives who suffer from hypertension, it's true that you yourself are at greater risk than others, but it does not mean that you will inevitably develop the disease. You can also counteract your increased risk through appropriate lifestyle measures. In three quarters of all hypertensive patients, a combination of lack of exercise and obesity is the primary cause, and in the remaining quarter, stress has a lot to do with high blood pressure. These are all factors you can influence!

High salt consumption

Salt used to be so precious it was used very sparingly, but today we consume it freely – not just because it has become dirt cheap, but also because salt has something to do with alertness. People with low blood pressure, who often feel tired and sluggish, can increase their blood pressure immediately and get themselves going with a cup of hot, salty broth.

But salt also has an effect on personal independence. Strange as it may sound, the more independent we human beings become, the more salt we consume. Primitive people who still have strong connections to the cosmos consume less than half a teaspoon of salt per day, and high blood pressure is unknown among them. In contrast, Western Europeans often swallow up to 15 g (almost 3 teaspoons) of salt per day without even trying. For most people, a low-salt diet containing a maximum of 6 g (1 teaspoon) per day tastes unbearably bland, but for salt-sensitive individuals (about half of all hypertensive patients!) it can help lower blood pressure by as much as 15 mmHg. You can test whether you're one of those people by eating a low-salt diet (see page 114) for a while and observing whether your blood pressure drops. Instead of salt, use plenty of fresh herbs for flavour.

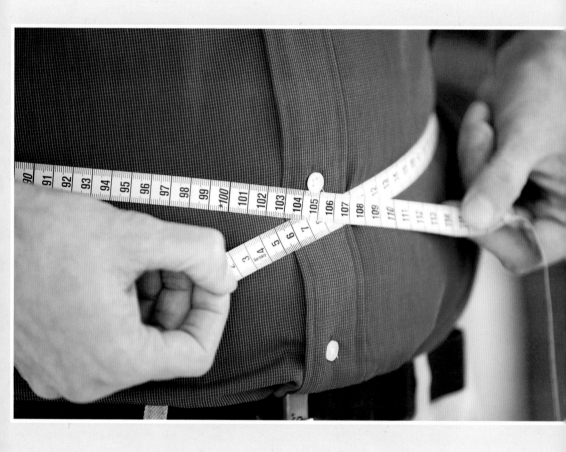

Constitution and Blood Pressure

Individual types

At birth, each person brings strengths, weaknesses, and unique traits into the world. Some people can eat whatever they want without getting fat, while others seem to put on weight simply by looking at food. Some people tend to be nervous; they get excited all the time and take every little detail personally. Others are unfazed by anything and keep their composure in the midst of chaos. These constitutional traits – whether bodily or psychological – are closely related to whether (and how) high blood pressure develops. People with high blood pressure can be assigned to one of three main groups according to their personal traits: the stress type, the abdominal type, and the chaos type. This is a way of recognising imbalances and taking advantage of them for therapeutic purposes. Your individual constitution is simply a foundation that is complemented by your lifestyle and personal circumstances. All these things combined can allow high blood pressure to develop.

The stress type

An estimated one-fifth of hypertensive patients belong to this type. They are usually slim; they're also usually perfectionists. These individuals are happy to accept responsibility (or have had responsibility forced on them by some stroke of destiny), but then they often expect too much of themselves, which eats away at their energy. They are thin-skinned and take every argument personally. On the other hand, they are also sensitive and empathetic and have a keen sense of what's essential. They have a great need to communicate and want to observe every emotion carefully, reflecting on it and analysing it. They tend to hide their light under a bushel and are seldom satisfied with themselves. They are easily made to feel insecure and then quickly become nervous and agitated. They tend to bottle up their anger and resentfulness, which they experience both as weakness and as a personal failure. Many of them allow their thoughts to revolve constantly around worries and problems and never find a way out, but are not open to receiving help.

Case studies

In this chapter and the next, you'll find examples of patients illustrating the concept of the three constitutional types. The cases are all real, but the names have been changed.

Case study 1: Claudia M.

Claudia M. is a 54-year-old widow with two grown-up daughters. For twenty years, she has been working as a bookkeeper for a large company, having worked her way up to that position with no formal training.

Her life has not always been easy. Her husband died of cancer when their daughters were ten and twelve, and she supported the family by herself. Meanwhile, the children have moved out of the house. For the past two years, Claudia has had a new young boss who keeps an eagle eye on all of her work and wonders out loud at least once a week whether this is really the right job for her. There's no doubt he wants to get rid of her – 'harassment' is the word that comes to mind – but she can't simply quit: lacking the appropriate professional credentials, she would not be able to find a comparable position anywhere else. Her boss's tactics are taking their toll: Claudia is barely able to relax any more, even at home at night. She sleeps poorly, not falling asleep until midnight even though she goes to bed at 10.30 pm at the latest. She wakes up around 3 am and feels as if she then stays awake until the alarm goes off in the morning. She arrives at work feeling exhausted and has difficulty concentrating. In just a few weeks, she loses almost nine pounds. She feels jittery, anxious, and thin-skinned and is often short of breath. Her heartbeat is very fast, with a resting pulse of about 100 beats per minute. Secretly checking her blood pressure at work, she finds it's consistently around 220/120 when she's at her desk – and not just after confrontations with the boss. During those clashes, her heart is in her mouth, her ears ring, her head pounds, and she feels dizzy and light-headed.

Claudia takes sick leave, but the boss has someone call her every day to make sure she's not just faking illness. Her primary care physician prescribes antihypertensive medications that are not totally effective. 24-hour monitoring shows that her blood pressure is often normal or even low during the day, with readings around 110/60 mmHg. Intermittently, however, it shoots up to around 220/120 and doesn't settle down to normal levels until she falls asleep. Meanwhile, Claudia has started taking sleeping pills at night, but they make her feel even drowsier in the morning. She's caught in a vicious cycle and sees no way out – until she finally finds a treatment that works. You'll learn about this treatment model on page 81.

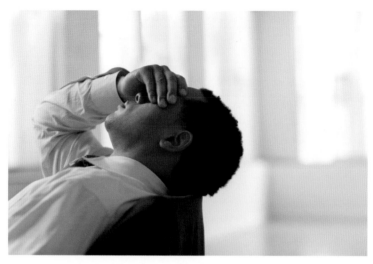

Persistent stress at work can drive up blood pressure.

Case study 2: Stefan B.

Stefan B. is 45 and married with three children. He loves his job and is comfortable in the school where he teaches. Not long ago, a colleague took sick leave and Stefan assumed responsibility for that class in addition to his own. He also became the chairman of the teachers' meeting and is involved in the school's remodeling and building project, which entails a lot of extra work. Often he gets home only between 9 and 10 pm. This has been going on for six months, and not without consequences. Stefan frequently wakes up feeling dizzy, light-headed, and not really present. He gets chilled easily and tends to have diarrhoea, which does his skinny body no good at all. During long days at school, it is not uncommon for him to feel his heart 'skip a beat'. Stefan is a perfectionist who does nothing half-heartedly, but he is becoming increasingly unable to live up to his own high expectations in class, in teachers' meetings, and in heading the construction process. At home, too, he is struggling to live up to the expectations of his wife, who also has a job, and his children complain that they almost never see their dad any more. Stefan feels 'burnt out' and empty, as if his life is living him instead of him shaping it. Blood pressure monitoring by his doctor results in some normal readings but also some around 180/95 mmHg. 24-hour monitoring reveals that those high figures are not just flukes; his blood pressure remains too high for longer periods of time. The diastolic (lower) figure in particular is often between 95 and 100. Stefan's blood pressure drops only during sleep. The signals are clear: something has to change in his life. On pages 83–84, you'll learn what Stefan decided to do.

Effects of stress

Two large studies have shown that stress can be a significant cause of high blood pressure. The CARDIA study followed 3,300 young men and women for fifteen years to investigate whether and how psychosocial stress affects blood pressure. The conclusion: the greater their impatience and feeling of being pressed for time, the more likely they were to develop high blood pressure. The Whitehall study, which involved 796 men between the ages of 35 and 55 and averaging 78 kilos (12 stone) in weight, investigated whether blood pressure rises during artificially induced stress situations and whether increased risk of developing high blood pressure could be deduced from such increases. The answer was a clear-cut 'yes'.

High demands and low control: a fatal combination

The examples of Claudia M. and Stefan B. demonstrate the disastrous effects of being pressed for time and under pressure at work while having little to no control over the situation. When individuals facing 'high demand' situations have little ability to influence those situations ('low control'), they feel helpless, angry, and afraid. Other examples include:

☞ Couriers and truck drivers on tight schedules. Every red light and traffic jam is a catastrophe for them.

☞ Office workers whose bosses constantly demand overtime while their families are waiting at home.

☞ Single parents juggling work and child-rearing responsibilities.

☞ Managers running companies which are threatened with closure or job cuts at the management level.

☞ Women experiencing gender discrimination.

The abdominal type

Abdominal types are the exact opposite of stress types. Their body type tends to be at least well-padded if not seriously overweight, and type 2 diabetes is not uncommon among them. They are habitually a bit lethargic, clumsy, and phlegmatic but are also deliberate, placid, and sociable. They are well buffered against stress of all sorts and are not easily thrown off track. At work and at home, they are solid as a rock – dependable, loyal, always there.

They are warm-hearted, empathetic, and sensitive. Physical activity is not their thing; they prefer to be couch potatoes. On the other hand, sensory pleasures mean a great deal to them: they enjoy good cooking and the taste of food is important to them. There are many variations of the abdominal type, depending on the cause of their excess weight, how satisfactorily they manage their professional and private life, and the intensity of their attitude toward life. Persistent stress can make even these generally thick-skinned people thin-skinned. They generally keep their feelings to themselves and bottle up negative emotions but tend to develop diarrhoea and shivering and start to panic quickly if such situations persist. In an attempt to become more thick-skinned again, they often eat when stressed, which drives their blood pressure back up – a fact they tend not to notice. Abdominal types barely perceive bodily signals because it is simply so difficult for souls to come to grips with such large bodies. That's why their blood pressure often remains elevated for many years without consequences.

Case study 3: Henry J.

Henry J. is 48 years old and divorced. He has two children who live with their mother. He thoroughly enjoys working as an art therapist, and his colleagues and patients alike are very appreciative of him and his work. Since his divorce three years ago, he lives alone in an apartment. His wife kept the house they had owned together and continues to live there with her new husband and the children. Henry is lonely now that he lives alone. Although deeply hurt that his wife preferred another man, he was both too kind and too lazy to want to fight to keep her. Henry has been drowning his sorrows in good food, and as a result he has gained 20 kilos (3 stone) in the past two years. He is 1.75 m tall (5 ft 8) and weighs almost 100 kilos (16 stone). Everything about him is well-padded, even his hands, although they look quite small in comparison to his big, heavy body. Henry is definitely not getting enough exercise. A walk once in a while? Well, OK,

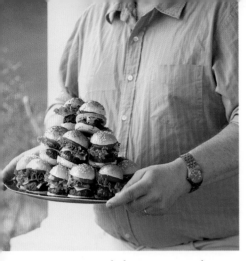

Homemade burgers are much tastier and healthier than ones from fast-food restaurants.

but nothing too athletic! He is becoming increasingly apathetic and slow, has a tremendous need for sleep, and struggles to get up in the morning. He often feels dizzy and light-headed before breakfast and becomes increasingly tired around 3 pm, even if he slept for ten hours the night before. Several cups of coffee are not enough to perk him up.

Henry's primary care physician has recorded very high blood pressure readings (190/100 mmHg), and prescription drugs have failed to lower his blood pressure. Long-term monitoring yields figures that remain consistently elevated throughout the day, dropping a bit only after a walk. Henry has stored up a lot of abdominal fat, and a glucose tolerance test indicates that his blood sugar levels are already elevated – the first stage of type 2 diabetes. Henry needs prompt intervention to prevent organ damage from high blood pressure and diabetes. You'll learn what his treatment model looks like on page 104.

Case study 4: Ricarda S.

Ricarda S. is 57 years old and has taken early retirement. She is married and has two grown-up children. Her ordeal began decades ago, when she suffered from severe postnatal depression after the birth of her twins. She has taken chemical antidepressants ever since. Later, digestive problems were added to her symptoms, and her doctor diagnosed irritable bowel syndrome. He increased her dosage of antidepressants several times, hoping they would help her summon up a bit of courage to face life, but she remains apathetic and generally goes about her work mechanically.

As a result of the high doses of antidepressants, Ricarda has gained huge amounts of weight, going from 68 to 130 kilos (11 stone to 20 stone) on a 1.65 m (5 ft 4) frame. She can barely move any more. Now that her doctor has also diagnosed diabetes and high blood pressure, Ricarda swallows a handful of pills every day. She is ashamed of her weight and feels responsible for her condition. Her daily life is more like dragging herself through the day than actually living, and she almost never leaves her apartment. She has long since lost confidence in medical science. There have been too many times when she was treated with disrespect, called a faker, or not taken seriously.

But Ricarda makes one final attempt when she comes across the address of the Herdecke Community Hospital on the internet. Turn to page 105 to find out what steps the doctors take and how Ricarda S. improves with their help.

Metabolic syndrome

What doctors call 'metabolic syndrome' consists of significant excess weight and abdominal fat along with high blood pressure, diabetes, and elevated triglycerides and low HDL cholesterol in the blood. Each of these factors is unhealthy on its own, and two or three in combination are enough to substantially increase the risk of cardiovascular disease.

The chaos type

People of this type have lost their rhythm on many levels and rarely manage to impose any structure on their life. They eat and sleep irregularly and all aspects of their life are erratic. They are irritable, unsatisfied, and nitpicking, but also have a gift for multitasking without losing their focus. Creativity is their great strength – they can make something out of any situation and get impatient when others can't keep up the pace. They are so active they can barely rest, and they are incapable of creating breaks for themselves. They are always burning the candle at both ends and often feel exhausted and burnt out. Their blood pressure is equally erratic and chaotic – sometimes too high, sometimes too low, especially when they have been prescribed antihypertensives because of sporadic high readings.

Case study 5: Manuela S.

This 36-year-old housewife is married and has three children, ages one, three and five. She is naturally thin-skinned and delicate. Although she is very intelligent and everything comes easily to her, she is unnerved by even minor difficulties and quickly becomes impatient and anxious.

These tendencies were exacerbated when she was pregnant with her youngest child: every little thing got on her nerves. She had morning sickness until the fifth month, which depleted her reserves. She felt ungrounded and driven by a mysterious inner restlessness, although there was no reason for it and everything was going smoothly at home. She did not understand what was going on with her and hoped that everything would be better once the baby was born.

She had a caring husband and help in the house, and the two little ones were bundles of joy and well-behaved. 24-hour blood pressure monitoring showed blood pressure rising sharply whenever she was especially agitated. She kept close watch on it in order to look out for possible gestational hypertension (see page 35) early, but this made her even more nervous, because she was afraid for herself and the baby. Everything went well, however, and the delivery was uncomplicated.

But now her agitation, instead of disappearing, is growing worse. Manuela is becoming even more restless, feels totally overwhelmed, and feels like she no longer sleeps at all. Four months after the birth, she weighs only 47 kilos (7 stone) at a height of 1.64 m (5 ft 4).

CONSTITUTION AND BLOOD PRESSURE

Manuela has become a stranger to herself. She is afraid because she doesn't know how to extricate herself from this situation. Her blood pressure continues to play tricks on her. It is sometimes extremely high, sometimes normal. But even at rest, her heartbeat is disproportionately fast at 90–120 beats per minute.

Turn to page 126 to find out how Manuela regained her centre.

Hypertensive crisis

When a chaos type's blood pressure goes up, it *really* goes up: readings of 230/120 mmHg are not uncommon. That's why people of this type are especially prone to hypertensive crises, which are often dangerous (see page 14).

Case study 6: Joseph B.

Joseph B. is a 55-year-old concert flautist. He is happily married with no children. For several years he has been at the peak of his artistic career: after a dry spell lasting for years, he is now a sought-after soloist giving performances all over the world. Although he travels a lot, he does not feel stressed – he loves his work and looks forward to every appearance.

Joseph is a very observant person. Not much escapes his attention. Although his wife has noticed times when he is completely exhausted, he himself is so wrapped up in his music that he seems unaware of it. For several weeks now, Joseph has been having frequent attacks of dizziness accompanied by a strange sensation of pressure in his head and very high blood pressure levels of around 230/120 mmHg, followed by normal readings of about 125/80. In the past year, he has gained 5 or 6 kilos (1 stone) and has the beginnings of a belly, which is certainly not uncommon

57

at his age; he is not even close to being obese. Joseph is not particular about food; he eats when he feels hungry, usually some sort of cold meal grabbed in a hurry. He can't remember the last time he sat down to a full, leisurely meal at a nicely set table.

Joseph is usually running from city to city and performance to performance and is seldom at home with his wife. Planes, taxis, hotels, concert halls – those are his points of reference. He has nowhere to retreat and rest. He sees the natural world only in passing and hasn't taken a walk in a long time. The sensory activities of seeing, smelling, tasting, and touching have receded completely into the background in comparison to hearing – music

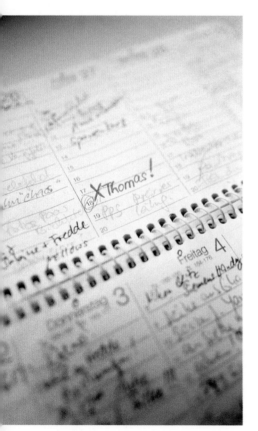

takes all his attention. Due to his packed calendar, he easily loses perspective, and he sleeps poorly and irregularly because of all the travelling and time changes. Once he has agreed to do a performance, he feels obliged to appear. Until recently, this creative chaos caused no problems for him – in fact, he enjoyed it and was comfortable with it – but now he notices it's often too much for him.

His primary care physician prescribes a beta blocker to reduce his blood pressure. It works, but the dizziness continues, and Joseph also notices heart palpitations before he falls asleep. Also, the medication affects his sexual potency, which makes him feel insecure. His self-image is getting shaky. He no longer knows who he is, which makes him anxious. As a result, his blood pressure goes up even more.

Chaos types often have a jam-packed diary and calendar.

58

Joseph knows that something has to change, but he has to make changes without endangering his career. See page 127 to learn how he managed to bring more rest and relaxation into his life.

Tranquility is the key to strength

This ancient bit of wisdom is especially true of people who travel a lot. For them, it's particularly important to have regularly scheduled islands of peace and relaxation so their bodies can regenerate.

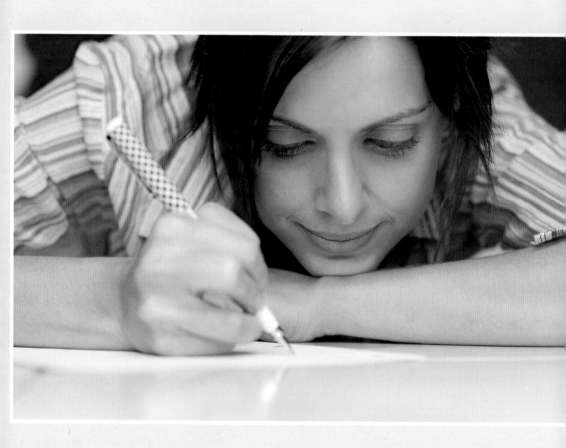

How to Determine Your Type

Which one are you: a stress type, an abdominal type, or a chaos type? It's important to find out so you can treat your high blood pressure type appropriately. The test on the following pages will help you do this.

Please don't cheat. Don't let your desire to have your test results avoid a certain type tempt you to provide false information. Each of the three types has favourable qualities, and each has its weaknesses. Be honest and true to yourself!

When scoring the test the first time, don't zero in on individual statements – on their own, they aren't indicative of type. Only your total score counts. The second time around, however, the individual statements will provide additional suggestions.

Test: which type are you?

Go through the following statements twice, marking the ones that apply to you.

The first time you go through the statements, consider which statements are definitely applicable to you (perhaps even familiar since adolescence)? Add up how often you answer with A, B, or C and record your totals on page 68. The frequency of your answers will determine whether you are primarily a stress, abdominal, or chaos type.

The second time you go through the statements, think about which statements are most applicable to you in the last two months. Select the five statements that currently have the most impact on your daily life.

How you feel

A. ☐ I feel my high blood pressure in the form of heart palpitations or pulsing in my throat.
B. ☐ I don't feel my high blood pressure at all.
A. ☐ I feel exactly what's going on in my body.
C. ☐ I've changed doctors umpteen times, but until my high blood pressure was discovered, nobody took me seriously.
A. ☐ My heart palpitations make me anxious.
B. ☐ I sleep like a log.
C. ☐ Always go to bed at the same time? Not me!
A. ☐ I have trouble falling asleep because there are still a thousand things running through my head.
C. ☐ I don't need much sleep.

B. ☐ I can sleep anywhere – even sitting up.

A. ☐ I often wake up in the middle of the night, especially after 2 a.m.

B. ☐ Sometimes I can hardly get out of bed in the morning.

A. ☐ When I'm stressed, I easily get headaches.

C. ☐ I've had frequent migraines for years.

A. ☐ I tend to have diarrhoea.

C. ☐ Regular bowel habits? Not me; sometimes I have diarrhoea, sometimes I'm constipated.

B. ☐ I get sweaty easily.

B. ☐ In bed, I'm a good substitute for a hot water bottle for my partner because I'm always warm.

B. ☐ I'm ashamed of being fat.

A. ☐ I often have cold hands and feet.

B. ☐ When I try to stick to a diet, I feel really miserable.

C. ☐ Life often seems to make no sense to me.

C. ☐ I'm afraid of the future even though things are going well for me and my family.

B. ☐ I don't see any meaning in life any more.

C. ☐ Other people are always worrying about me and it gets on my nerves.

Blood pressure

A. ☐ The only things that make my blood pressure go up are excitement, exertion, and arguments. Other than that, it's normal.

B. ☐ My blood pressure has gone up only since I've gained so much weight.

C. ☐ I've never checked my blood pressure before. What for?

A. ☐ In the doctor's office, my blood pressure is normal, but when I check it at home, it's often too high (or vice versa).

B. ☐ If you check your blood pressure all the time, you'll just drive yourself crazy.

C. ☐ My blood pressure varies a lot and I can't explain it.

A. ☐ It's especially the lower figure that's elevated; it's usually not below 90. When I get worried and check again, the readings are usually even higher and my pulse rate is over 100.

B. ☐ I can't possibly have high blood pressure – I'm always relaxed!

C. ☐ My blood pressure always goes down again, so why should I take pills?

Food and drink

B. ☑ I've always enjoyed cooking and eating.

C. ☐ It makes no difference to me whether I eat fast food or gourmet food. Taste isn't that important.

C. ☐ All those cooking shows on TV – why so much fuss about food?

A. ☐ Eating isn't that important to me.

C. ☐ I often forget to eat.

A. ☐ I'm not a breakfast person. I can't eat before 10 am.

A. ☐ I like to have breakfast late and then eat something hot.

C. ☐ I need several cups of coffee a day – espresso is best, black and hot.

A. ☐ Coffee doesn't agree with me. It makes no difference whether it's espresso, latte, or just regular coffee.

A. ☐ Hot chocolate with whipped cream really warms me up.

C. ☐ I appreciate good wine.

B. ☐ I sometimes like to have one drink too many.

B. ☐ There's nothing better than a ham hock with dumplings.

A. ☐ Lunch always has to be a quick meal for me.

C. ☐ Go out to eat? When would I have time? I can hardly enjoy it, anyway.

B. ☐ I always need something to munch on in between meals.

A. ☐ I love chocolate and cake.

B. ☐ Cake just doesn't taste good without whipped cream.

C. ☐ Even when I was a kid, my mother said I ate like a little bird.

A. ☐ When I'm under stress, I tend to lose weight instead of gaining it.

B. ☐ When I'm feeling stressed, I have to eat.

A. ☐ When I'm upset, I can't eat anything.

B. ☐ Whenever I'm sad, I need something sweet.

C. ☐ There are many foods I just can't digest.

B. ☐ Plump people are happier.

C. ☐ There are so many environmental contaminants in foods these days. I have to be careful not to eat the wrong thing.

B. ☐ It used to be easy for me to lose a few kilos/pounds, but it's harder now that I'm older.

B. ☐ I've already tried lots of diets and none of them did any good.

Habits and behaviour

A. ☐ It's hard for me to sit still.

C. ☑ It's hard for me to unwind.

B. ☐ I stay calm when others are getting nervous.

C. ☐ I'm not good at maintaining order.

B. ☐ I enjoy being lazy.

C. ☐ I love creative chaos.

A. ☐ It's hard for me to say no.

C. ☐ I'm good at improvising.

A. ☐ I'm really good at organising.

C. ☐ Organising and delegating are difficult for me.

C. ☐ I like to take charge of everything that's going on around me.

B. ☐ Other people always think they can do whatever they want with me, but there *are* limits to my patience and ability to work under pressure.

C. ☐ I'm the only one who can find anything on my desk.

A. ☐ My day is well-planned, but something always intervenes.

C. ☐ I'm often late.

B. ☐ When I have free time, I love doing nothing!

B. ☐ I often don't feel like doing anything and would just as soon take it easy at home.

C. ☐ In the evening I often wonder why I didn't accomplish what I intended to do – again!

C. ☐ I'm not particular about when I go to bed (usually late).

B. ☐ I enjoy watching sports on television. Anything as long as I don't have to do it myself!

B. ☐ Exercise is murder.

C. ☐ I enjoy travelling.

B. ☐ I don't like climbing stairs because I always get out of breath.

B. ☐ I always take the car to run errands – isn't that what we have it for?

A. ☐ Even when I'm on holiday, I want to be active – just lying on the beach is not my thing.

B. ☐ My hobbies and clubs are very important to me.

B. ☐ I feel best with my family and friends around me.

A. ☐ Arguing doesn't agree with me. It stays with me for hours afterward and I have a hard time getting away from it.

B. ☐ I may be laid-back, but I'm still thin-skinned.

A. ☐ I'm aware of any tension in the room. If someone doesn't trust me, I notice immediately.

A. ☐ I take criticism very personally.

A. ☐ When I'm angry, I prefer to keep my mouth shut. There's not much else I can do.

B. ☐ I see everything that's going on but prefer to keep it to myself.

B. ☐ It pains me when people make fun of my weight, but I don't let it show.

A. ☐ I prefer to deal with problems on my own.

B. ☐ Talking is not my thing; I'm not a person of many words.

A. ☐ I would have a lot to say, but nobody listens to me.

A. ☐ I'm not good at talking about feelings, and most people don't understand what I mean anyway.

A. ☐ I hate pity.

C. ☐ I can't stand pedantic people.

C. ☐ I don't really feel at home anywhere.

Job and relationship

A. ☐ At work I have to do whatever my boss demands.

A. ☐ My boss will not tolerate being contradicted.

C. ☐ I am not a good boss.

A. ☐ I'm not interested in elbowing my way up at work.

B. ☐ At work, I'm the one who always has to cover for my colleagues.

C. ☐ I often feel overwhelmed by it all.

A. ☐ I'd prefer to work as a team, but it's a real free-for-all here. It's everyone for him or herself.

B. ☐ My colleagues appreciate my dependability.

C. ☐ When there are problems at work, I immediately feel panicky.

C. ☐ Independence is important to me.

A. ☐ There's no one I can talk to about my problems.

C. ☐ My partner often tells me not to make such a fuss.

C. ☐ My rule of thumb in my relationship is to know when to shut up.

A. ☐ My partner is very authoritarian and always has to be right.

C. ☐ Conflict with my partner is hard on me. I need harmony.

B. ☐ I'm not eating any more since my partner left me, but I'm gaining weight steadily.

A. ☐ My partner is the one who wears the trousers in our house. What he/she says, goes.

B. ☐ In my relationship, loyalty and dependability are important to me.

Scoring

First round results:

> Number of A answers __
> Number of B answers __
> Number of C answers __

If A is your most frequent answer, you're a stress type.

If B is your most frequent answer, you're an abdominal type.

If C is your most frequent answer, you're a chaos type.

Most people are a mixture of all three types, with emphasis on one. You can select the appropriate components to put together your treatment programme.

Second round results:

My top five statements for the last two months are:

1. _____

2. _____

3. _____

4. _____

5. _____

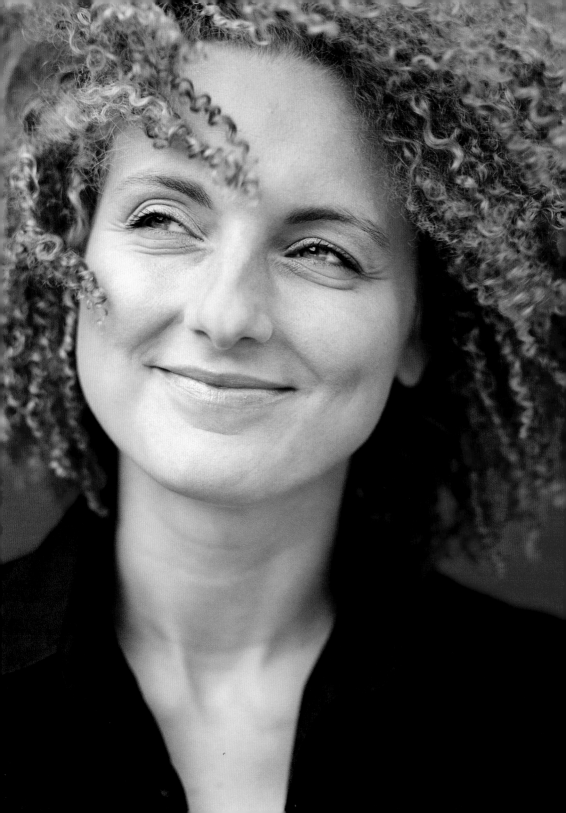

PART TWO
Practice

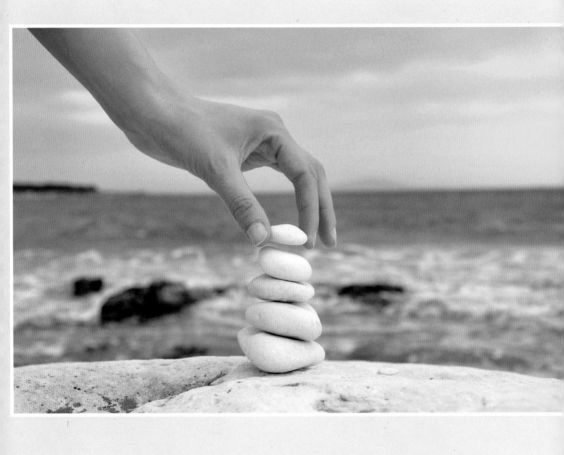

The Building Blocks of Well-being

In this chapter, you'll learn about a type-oriented programme that aims to help you not only normalise your blood pressure but also feel better and enjoy life more. The more you *enjoy* tackling your high blood pressure, the better it will work. And the more you feel better in general, the easier it will be for you to change one or more aspects of your daily life. So get motivated!

The great thing about this programme is that it's fun. You don't have to give up cake or coffee or that Sunday roast. And if you don't want to go to the gym or go jogging every morning, we understand! Instead, you can select from a full spectrum of possible measures that are appropriate for your type and will work better in *your* daily life.

Our intention is not to make you fearful or threaten you with the possibility of illness or even early death if you don't follow these suggestions. Risk analysis based purely on statistics is not what we have in mind either. Dwelling on potential risks is no way to develop motivation. Most people won't eat differently or get more exercise simply to reduce their risk of heart attack or stroke ten years from now, but they will happily continue once they see lifestyle changes lead to greater energy, endurance, and enjoyment of life within just a few weeks. This is how we want to motivate you and help you focus on yourself. Your individual case may not be reflected in any statistics but is all-important in finding effective treatment for you. We want to encourage you to discover the predispositions and situations that drive your blood pressure up and to provide you with tools for recognising changes in your life that will make you feel well. And these changes will also reduce your risk of cardiovascular disease.

Treatment for high blood pressure is often strictly oriented towards getting the numbers down. However, blood pressure readings are just snapshots – with the exception of 24-hour monitoring (see page 37). In addition, high blood pressure can be high for many very different reasons. The determining factors in an abdominal type are different from those in a stress type, and these differences also influence treatment. This means that in every case, hypertensive therapy must take the individual's constitution into account – not just their recorded levels.

Only half of all hypertensive patients take their medication

Repeated studies have shown that almost half of all patients with hypertension fail to take their prescription medication as directed. Some people simply forget to take the tablets in the absence of any acute symptoms, but in most cases they experience side effects severe enough to persuade them not to take their pills or to take lower or less frequent doses. What's going on here? One crucial reason may well be that doctors almost never take the patient's constitution and life situation into account in selecting medications. In fact, they are usually unaware of factors they ought to be considering and are simply following the guidelines established by professional associations more or less blindly. Other approaches are certainly possible, however, even if the guidelines are followed. You will learn how on page 143.

Your actions are more important than you think

High blood pressure is not a stroke of fate that appears out of the clear blue sky. It always results from a combination of constitution and lifestyle. This combination must also be the starting point for treatment – and the most important player in this process is you! Only you can influence these two factors. You can counteract your type's inherent imbalances, and if your lifestyle promotes high blood pressure, you can make changes so your body no longer has any reason to drive your blood pressure up.

It's up to you!

Of course drugs can lower your blood pressure, but you can also lower it yourself. Even more importantly, you can do it with fewer side effects. And the great thing about it is that you'll enjoy life so much more!

What is crucial here are your intentions and your actions. If you make no lifestyle changes but simply depend on drugs to do the work, there will be no change in the factors that caused your blood pressure to go up in the

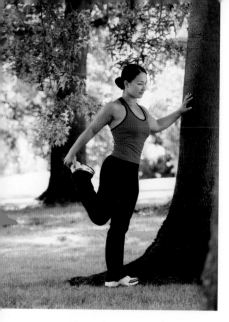

Physical activity is important in treating high blood pressure.

first place. In the long run, only steps you take yourself will eliminate the reasons for it, and the most important thing is to enjoy taking these steps. Don't just simply follow your doctor's directions to the letter. You will need to understand why something needs to change in your life and actively help make it happen.

Hypertensive treatment must always address both body and soul because their intersection is where blood pressure develops. It's always essential to restore balance between life's polarities. Health is not the absence of disease but the daily activity of finding a middle ground in the alternation between activity and rest, waking and sleeping, working and relaxing, outside and inside, breaking down and building up. This balance is highly individual. Only you can discover what you need in order to achieve it – and that's why we have developed this programmeme. You can tailor it to your own needs, selecting combinations that correspond best to your individual situation. It's a modular system that you adapt to changing circumstances in your life. That's why it's so universal and applicable to any stage of life.

A tailored programme

Our type-oriented programme of action takes your capabilities into account and can be adapted for any type in any life situation. High blood pressure, after all, is only a sign that you have a weakness somewhere that needs to be balanced out. If that is done successfully, your body no longer has any reason to drive your blood pressure up. And one nice side effect is that you will feel better and more energetic in general. You'll enjoy life more and remain healthier in the long run. Drugs do have a place in this process, but the basis for prescribing them should be specific individual needs, not the abstract statistical findings of studies (see page 143). The entire programme is based on a choice of ways to tackle the most important factors influencing your blood pressure: your daily schedule, physical activity, nutrition, personal hygiene, and psychological balance. You can combine these 'building blocks' as needed to restore your blood pressure's natural, healthy variability, to achieve a balanced relationship between rest and activity, to balance out opposites, and to bring harmony to your life. They will also help you in your efforts to eat healthy, tasty food; bring rhythm into your day; recognise your body's signals and listen to your inner voice; and be creative and take responsibility for what you do.

Putting together your programme

Look for all the steps that correspond to your type (stress, abdominal or chaos) and your current situation and write them on a piece of paper.

Select from these options according to your own preferences. In other words, your choices should be based on what you'll enjoy. They shouldn't be based on anything you're afraid of. Be realistic and don't expect too much of yourself. Trying to change everything at once is a recipe for failure.

Consider your options: which changes do you want to implement for the long term, either daily or on certain days of the week? Which ones will you implement for a limited time, say, the next three or six months?

Review your choices every so often to see what you need at the moment and what steps might serve that purpose. You'll always find an appropriate combination of 'building blocks'.

What if you don't belong to one single type?

Sometimes our test fails to yield a clear-cut result and you can't really assign yourself to any one of the three types. But you can still use our programme to good advantage.

Think about these things: what are the characteristics that have most actively shaped your life until now? Which of the three types is most characteristic of you? Which of the types do you recognise as being most like you? That one is your basic type.

What has happened in the last few weeks or months that is having a lasting influence on your life? Ask yourself which situations are most like yours.

This will give you a basis for recognising which characteristics you have. You can then look for long-term steps to take in the coming year and turn into habits. In addition, choose suggestions from the other lists of options that address your situation.

Here's an example: you are basically an abdominal type, but for several months now you've been experiencing increased stress at work, which is making you nervous and disturbing your sleep. As a result, you've been enjoying the distraction and numbing effect of a couple glasses of wine or beer in the evenings. In this case, you should select your long-term steps from the list for abdominal types and supplement them with building blocks for stress types until the situation at work calms down. This is an example of how therapeutic measures to improve your high blood pressure can be adapted to changing circumstances in our life without becoming any less effective. One more important tip: stress and abdominal types are characterised by obvious one-sided traits. Chaos types, however, are not – their most obvious characteristic is an inability to achieve balance. To a certain extent, this is also true of stress and abdominal types. So all the suggestions we provide for chaos types are also helpful for the two other types. All of them strengthen your centre and are fundamentally health-promoting.

Yes, you can!

In 2008, the motto of Barack Obama, then candidate for President of the US, resonated around the world, and it applies to you, too: yes, you can! In the beginning, some of our suggestions will sound like drudgery, but don't let that discourage you. The nice thing about this programme is that success comes quickly. After just one week, you'll feel like something is missing if you haven't been outside in the fresh air. You'll notice that you suddenly get more done when you plan your day well, or that your inner restlessness disappears when you spend ten minutes meditating in the evening and consciously let your day end peacefully. And almost coincidentally, you'll notice that your blood pressure is normalising.

No drug in the world can duplicate successful experiences like this – only you can make them happen for yourself. Everything you do, you do for yourself – for your quality of life, for your health, for your very personal, individual well-being. Yes, you can!

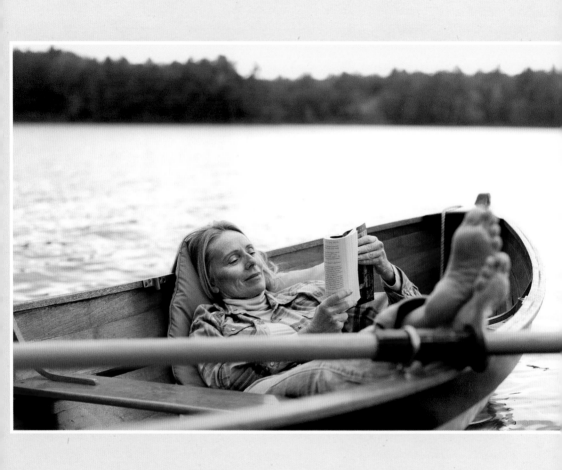

The Programme for Stress Types

If you're always running on adrenalin or you get nervous at the slightest provocation, the programme that follows is just right for you. It is designed to bring more calmness into your life and to make you more grounded and thick-skinned. But it can also help you relax your standards of perfection and loosen up a bit. In this chapter, you will learn the basics of how to go about it.

Successful treatment plans

First, though, we want to reveal the treatment plans for the two patients we introduced in the last chapter. These two examples will show you how different stress types can be ... and how their treatment can be individualised.

Case study 1: Claudia M

Claudia M. (see page 48) comes to the Herdecke Community Hospital for in-patient treatment. An ultrasound of her heart reveals some thickening of the left ventricle wall – already a consequence of long-term elevated blood pressure and a sign of early-stage cardiac insufficiency. Checking her blood pressure always makes Claudia anxious: her individual readings are mostly 20mmHg higher than in 24-hour monitoring. To avoid overdosing or underdosing her, the doctor adjusts her medication, discontinuing the calcium antagonist prescribed by her primary care physician and keeping an ACE inhibitor in combination with a diuretic (see page 144). Several anthroposophical medications (see page 147) are added: Aurum/Hyoscyamus comp. taken as drops during the day and by subcutaneous injection above the navel at night; Plumbum mellitum D20 in powder form three times a day; and Bryophyllum mother tincture (drops) three times a day. In addition, Claudia's feet are rubbed with lavender oil in the evening and she receives painting therapy and curative eurythmy (see page 161) once a day. After a week, her blood pressure readings even out during the day. She feels tired but relaxed. She is still not sleeping well, however, and wakes up regularly between 2 am and 4 am in the morning, so her evening injection of Aurum/Hyoscyamus is discontinued and replaced with Hyoscyamus/Valeriana drops. In case she wakes up during the night, the doctor recommends taking the Hyoscyamus/Valeriana drops again, then eating a spoonful of honey and putting on wool socks so her feet stay warm. Claudia sets everything she needs for this ritual out on the nightstand, and in fact it works. It usually takes no more than fifteen minutes before she falls asleep again.

Each morning, Claudia gets a full-body rub-down with sea salt (see page 121) and lemon bath milk. In addition, a lemon is squeezed directly into the wash water to add its etheric oils.

By now she is feeling much better, has gained 2 kilos (half a stone), and has plucked up new courage to face her life. She is also determined to stand up to harassment at work. She has decided not to answer the phone when she sees her boss is calling and to look around for a good employment lawyer. A course of mind-body therapy will help support the progress she has made.

Repeating the 24-hour monitoring reveals that her blood pressure rises no higher than 140 mmHg during the day. As a result, the combination drug she has been taking can be traded in for an ACE inhibitor alone.

Holistic treatment

It's important to tackle high blood pressure on multiple levels at the same time, and medications are also selected according to this principle.

Case study 2: Stefan B

For Stefan B. (see page 50), the first priority is to help him regain his energy, so he takes a nourishing bath with cream (see box overleaf) three times a week. Nothing about the situation at school can change in the five months remaining until the summer holidays, so Stefan needs to structure his day rhythmically, because rhythm is energising. Every three hours, he takes a ten-minute break for a mindfulness exercise (see page 101) to switch his head off and his senses on. This gives him time to collect himself instead of rushing from one task to the next. Whenever he can fit it in, either at noon or in the course of the afternoon, he goes home for a brief nap and then returns to school. To feel calmer in the evening, he reviews the day in reverse (see page 139) shortly before going to bed. After the summer holidays, his responsibilities at work will be reduced; he will be able to give up the responsibility for the teachers' conference and the new building and concentrate fully on working with his class, which will be much more manageable. To support his cardiovascular function, Stefan takes three anthroposophical medications every day (see page 148): Neurodoron, Bryophyllum tincture, and Cardiodoron. They allow him to maintain his blood pressure at around 140/90mmHg and to dispense with conventional drugs.

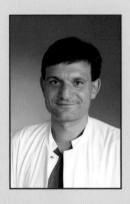

My personal tip

Nourishing cream baths

This bath is ideal when overwork and stress have exhausted your body. Here's how to do it: whisk ½ litre (1 pint) of milk or cream together with an egg and pour the mixture into warm bath water, stirring to form a milky/creamy emulsion. Scoop out one litre in a bowl, cut an organic lemon in half, and use the bottom of a glass to press both halves out under water in the bowl. Add the lemon water to the bath, relax in the tub for about 20 minutes, and hop into your snug, pre-warmed bed as soon as you get out.

A nourishing bath in the evening stimulates the whole body via the skin and encourages nutrient storage. The very next morning, you'll feel stronger and ready for a hearty breakfast, which will also nourish and strengthen you.

Notice your body's signals

Stress types tend to ask too much of themselves all the time – a sure way to drive blood pressure up. So taking the time to sense whether you've overstepped your limits again is a very beneficial exercise: shouldn't you take a break at some point? Isn't it long past bedtime? When you consciously observe your body's signs of exhaustion, you'll find your blood pressure no longer goes up so much.

Developing a mindful lifestyle

People who belong to the stress type often lead hectic lives. As they become increasingly hyperactive and nervous, they run themselves ragged emotionally. They need effective ways to calm down at intervals throughout the day.

Take a break

Studies show that we cannot work with full concentration for longer than an hour and a half at a stretch. Our attention invariably wanders – unless, that is, we take a short break and then a longer one every three hours. That's why the daily schedule in many cloisters and monasteries is arranged in short blocks – throughout the day, the bell rings to call the monks and nuns to prayer (see page 21). A culture that includes time

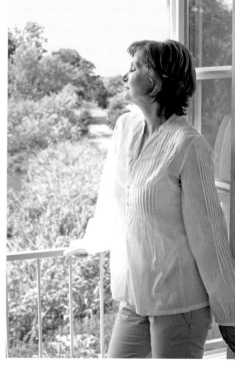

To clear your head, open the window and take a deep breath!

85

to 'exhale' provides opportunities for reflection after the 'inhaling' period of active work. This rhythm supports responsiveness and flexibility in all body functions, especially blood pressure.

Reduce the pressure

If, like many stress types, you have been under extreme pressure for a long time, it's essential to take a close look at what is causing the pressure. What is hemming you in? What can't you say no to? When you're constantly repressing pent-up aggression, your blood pressure invariably goes up. Stress of this sort is most dangerous when coupled with a feeling of impotence and helplessness: your body pumps out increased quantities of stress hormones, which keep your blood pressure elevated and make your heart beat faster. It's like running a car's engine at full speed until it finally overheats and just stops. Don't let it get to that point.

Look for opportunities to vent your frustrations – out in the woods, where you can just let loose and scream without disturbing anyone, or on the playing field where you can work out your aggressions.

Find someone to help you analyse everything that weighs you down and all the injustices you experience. It feels good to discuss these things with someone you trust, someone who is not involved in the problem and can see it from a totally different perspective.

If needed, don't hesitate to seek professional help, too – from a helpline, a psychologist, or a psychotherapist.

At work, think about which problems require immediate solutions. Where do you need to push back to avoid adverse consequences to yourself? Perhaps you need legal help or arbitration. You can also approach the workers' council or your union. Or is it time to think about retraining?

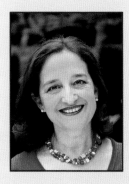

My personal tip

Renewed energy in two minutes

Deliberately taking breaks preserves your energy and calms you down, so you should fit in a break roughly every 90 minutes, even if it's just for two minutes. What to do during your break?

☞ Open the window and take ten deep breaths, blowing hard as you breathe out.

☞ Splash your face with cold water or spray on some facial toner.

☞ Stand at the door and open your senses wide: what does it smell like here? What is there to hear?

☞ Stand up and stretch. Pull your shoulders down and back to open up your ribcage. Inhale and exhale deeply.

☞ Make a cup of tea or do part of the preparation for lunch or dinner (do a bit more in your next break).

You'll see – you'll end these short breaks feeling refreshed. You'll be ready to concentrate again and focus on new activities.

In your private life, for relationship problems, you can seek help from a mediator. Church or community organisations can help you find one. Mediators are trained to help people in conflict arrive at compromises without involving the courts. Apply for respite care if parenting responsibilities or daily stressors are getting to be too much for you.

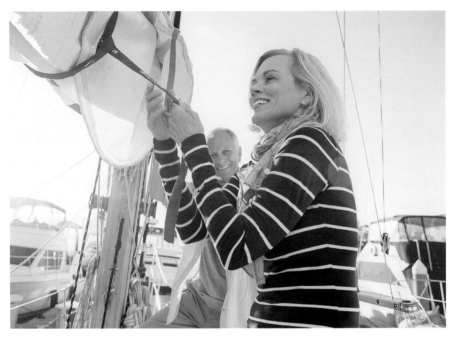

Sailing is a great sport for fitness and relaxation – especially for people under stress.

Don't be afraid of change – where one door closes, another opens. The current crisis may already hold the seeds of a better future.

Enjoy your evenings

Don't just fall into bed exhausted – that just allows the day's experiences to keep on driving you, making it hard for you to fall asleep. It makes much more sense to end the day in a gentle fashion.

☞ Have a quiet supper, preferably with your family or partner, but you can make the meal pleasant even if you live alone: light a candle on the table and use a decorative place mat and a nice place setting. You eat with your eyes, too!

☞ Go for a walk, even if it's just for five minutes or around the garden.

☞ Limit TV viewing and read a few pages in a good book or listen to your favourite music.

☞ Make a habit of leaving the day behind you. Look back over the day or write a few sentences in your diary.

☞ If you still have trouble falling asleep, take a spoonful of honey 15–30 minutes before going to bed. You can either take it straight or stir it into tea or warm milk.

☞ Get enough sleep. Go to bed before midnight. The next morning, you'll notice immediately that you're more rested, calmer, and more ready for action.

Create an oasis of enjoyment

Even in the midst of crisis, no matter how tyrannical your boss or resentful your colleagues, there are still things you can do to help you feel more content. Create a little oasis of quiet enjoyment, a 'garden' that only you can access and that you can enjoy briefly each day. Put a flower, a postcard, or a photo on the desk or hang a picture on the wall – one that you really like and that gives you a feeling of calmness and confidence. Whenever the stress gets to be too much, look at the picture, take a deep breath, and know that no one can take this enjoyment away from you. And don't neglect your desk! Keep it clean and leave it tidy every night. If possible, arrange the furniture so you have a nice view.

Type-appropriate nutrition

Stress types tend not to care too much about food. They're more likely to stuff down a quick bite when they can. No wonder their blood pressure doesn't co-operate, if their bodies aren't properly nourished! The antidote to this is simple: it's called 'meal time'. It's part of the culture of taking breaks and helps you get out of your habitual daily grind.

Eat oats for energy

Rolled oats – in the form of muesli or warm oatmeal, for example – are ideal for breakfast or as a between-meal snack. Oats are rich in magnesium and phosphorus, so they give you a real shot of energy. That's why horses are given plenty of oats to prepare them for peak performance. For human stress types, an oat-rich snack can help recharge your batteries quickly.

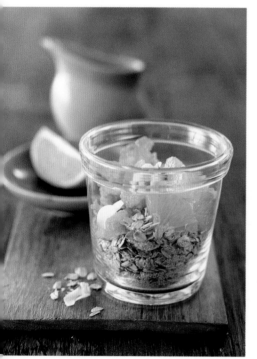

Oats are a tasty source of energy.

Have a good breakfast

Don't start your day by dashing out of the house because you got up late again. Two or three hours later, you'll be starving, but by then you'll be in the thick of it at work with no time to eat. You make do by grabbing something quick to eat, but you're still stuck in the same rut. Approach your day deliberately, right from the start. Even if you have very little time in the morning or just aren't a breakfast person, you can sit down for five or ten minutes and have a bite to eat. You'll enjoy the feeling of well-being it brings – and already you'll be approaching your day differently. Your blood sugar won't drop as quickly, either, especially if you can fit in a mid-morning snack before lunch. Here are a few suggestions for quick, nourishing breakfasts:

Roasted oats

Ingredients:
  50 g (¼ cup) butter, 100 g (1 cup) rolled oats (i.e., not quick-cooking or instant), two tablespoons of sugar.

Preparation:
  Heat the butter in a frying pan over high heat
  Add the oats and sugar and stir
  Keep stirring until the oats are brown
  Be careful – the time between 'done' and 'burnt' is extremely short!

Variations: roast pine nuts or flax, sunflower, or pumpkin seeds along with the oats.

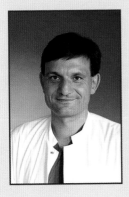

My personal tip

Drink beetroot juice!

Three or four hours after drinking ½ litre (1 pint) of beetroot juice, your systolic blood pressure (upper number) drops by 10 mmHg and the diastolic (lower) figure by 8 mmHg ... and the effect lasts for up to 23 hours! This was proven by a study conducted at the London School of Medicine.

Nutritious snacks

Sometimes stressful situations that make you nervous and drive your blood pressure up don't occur until several hours after one of your main meals. When this happens, make sure to have a snack that will help give you energy (and remind you to take a break!) For your snack break, don't choose fast food or a chocolate bar – they'll just make your blood sugar skyrocket and then drop just as fast. More nutritious, easily digestible snacks include rice cakes, fruit, nuts, trail mix, or dried fruit. Vegetable broth or miso soup (find it in Oriental food stores) is pleasantly warming and makes you feel comfortably full. A piece of dark chocolate (50–70% cacao content) will also satisfy acute hunger and even lower your blood pressure (upper figure) by about 5 mmHg without provoking fears of weight gain. (Milk chocolate doesn't have the same effect.) Instead of coffee, it's better to drink tea, which is less stimulating, or – better still – ginger water, herbal tea, or a fruit juice spritzer.

Eat mindfully

Don't do anything else while you eat – no reading the newspaper, answering emails, or looking at your laptop. All the flavours will be much more pronounced if you concentrate totally on your food.

You eat with your eyes, too!

Cultivate these good eating habits:

☞ *Always* sit down to eat. That means no eating standing up or while heading out the door of the office. If you're driving, unpack your sandwich once you get to the car park instead of polishing it off during the drive. And that kebab you grab for a snack? You'll be more comfortable eating it sitting down.

☞ If you absolutely have to eat at your desk, put the papers aside, spread out a big cloth napkin, set out a ceramic plate and a glass of water (or tea or juice) and light a candle. Don't eat anything straight from the package, but arrange the food nicely on the plate.

☞ Sit quietly for a moment while you take in this sight, take a couple of deep breaths, remind yourself to enjoy the meal – and only then begin eating.

☞ If you apply these tips, you will find yourself eating with pleasure instead of hastily shovelling in your food. Eating more slowly warms not only your stomach but also your heart. If you chew slowly and deliberately and really taste what you're eating, you'll feel a comfortable sensation of fullness.

Eat easily digestible food

Rich, heavy food doesn't agree with nervous people, so your meals should be light and easily digestible. Don't give your gut too much work to do, or it will rebel with cramps, pain, flatulence, or diarrhoea. Still, your food must also contain enough nutrients to provide your body with the energy it needs.

☞ Avoid raw food – it spends too much time in your stomach and intestines. Instead, cook your vegetables: steaming until they're crisp-tender makes them more digestible. Choose wholegrain products, but make sure the grain is finely ground. Coarse grains are too much work for your intestines.

☞ Don't hesitate to eat meat or fish more frequently, but pay attention to good quality and sustainable practice. The high protein content of dairy products also makes them appropriate for you to consume daily, because protein-rich food is easier to digest. All types of soups are also good because they're warming and therefore relaxing, especially in the evening.

☞ Eating smaller portions throughout the day rather than two or three big meals is easier on your digestive tract, while still providing adequate nourishment.

☞ If you are a salt-sensitive individual, choose low-salt foods (see page 114).

Wholegrain, but easily digestible

Wholegrain products that leave the grains intact are not easy to digest – the coarse texture is too rough on your digestive tract. Instead, choose products made from whole kernels that have been finely ground, such as whole-grain semolina or corn grits. They can be used in both savoury recipes (like soups and veggie burgers) and sweet ones (porridge, puddings), and the fine grind will give you the full benefit of the nutrients.

Exercise and physical activity

The exercise programme for stress types is more recreational than athletic. The point is not to make you burn calories, since you probably don't have any extra meat on your bones. Instead, the priority is to get you off the treadmill of your daily life and (preferably) out into the fresh air, where you should take the opportunity to relax rather than stressing yourself further with athletic ambitions. Movement should create a comfortable sensation of warmth and make you feel pleasantly tired but definitely not exhausted. Any type of movement that makes you slow down and get centred is good for you.

☞ Going for walks is easy, and you can do it anywhere and for free! As you walk, open up all your senses: what does it smell like outside?

What's that I'm hearing? What does the landscape look like? What colour is the sky? How are the clouds moving? Do you feel the wind on your skin and the sun or raindrops on your face?

☞ Every so often, plan an outing that includes a short hike followed by stopping for a bite to eat. Or stimulate all your senses and work up an appetite by taking a walk on the beach and feeling the wind whipping around your ears.

☞ Archery is especially good for concentration because you have to focus on the essentials.

☞ If you enjoy dancing, try learning to tango. You can't let your mind wander, or you won't connect with your dance partner.

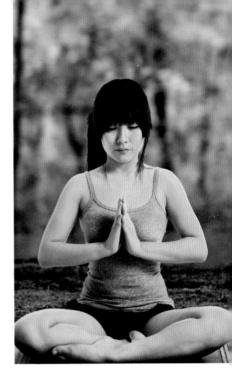

Yoga outdoors is ideal for stress types.

☞ Tai chi, qi gong, and yoga are all highly recommended for stress types, as are golf, horseback riding, sailing, biking, badminton, and volleyball.

Good for your body

Massages are a wonderful way to relax. Get your partner to give you a massage or treat yourself to a professional massage once a week. There are many types of relaxing massages; we recommend them all, almost without exception. Submitting to warm, gently circling hands is enough to bring you to peace all by itself. We especially recommend sound massages, in which singing bowls that vibrate at different frequencies are placed on the body. Their sound not only fills the whole room but is also transmitted to your entire body, making you feel balanced and peaceful.

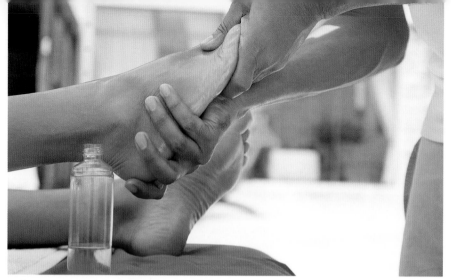

A foot massage with lavender oil is instantly refreshing and relaxing for stress types.

When there isn't time for a full body or back massage, a foot rub before going to sleep helps pull everything that got stuck in your head in the course of the day down into your feet and out. It's incredible how easily you'll fall asleep after – or sometimes even during – your foot rub. It's really simple to do: rub a few drops of oil or foot cream between your hands and spread it over the back and sole of the foot with gentle pressure. Your thumbs can press the arch of the foot upward while your fingers glide over the middle of the foot. To finish, pull gently on each toe in succession and stroke the whole foot with both hands again. That's how to give yourself a foot massage if there's no one around to do it for you. Afterward, put on fuzzy wool socks and slip into bed right away. You will fall asleep quickly!

Lavender, rose, and juniper oils are especially good for stress types. Lavender is calming and relaxing, rose is enveloping and protective, and juniper is strengthening. But it's also perfectly all right to choose a different oil if you prefer its scent. The important thing is to use only good quality, additive-free massage oils. Before you buy, make sure that your choice contains only etheric oils from natural sources – ideally, from wild-crafted plants – rather than synthetics.

Stay nice and warm

In stress types, warmth often gets dammed up in the head, while hands and feet tend to be cold. Here's how to counteract this tendency:

☞ Make sure your hands and feet stay warm by wearing gloves, wool socks, slippers, and clothing with cuffs at the wrists and ankles.

☞ Have a warm drink between meals, such as a cup of freshly brewed herbal tea, hot ginger water with a spoonful of honey, or hot lemon and honey.

☞ Wear a muff when you walk outside in winter. On cold days, it keeps your hands much warmer than gloves.

☞ Before going to bed, take a warm bath, preferably with lavender bath oil, so you will be warm and relaxed when you slip under the covers.

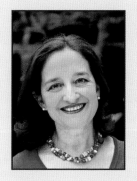

My personal tip
Add juniper oil to your bath

Etheric oil of juniper is hard to find, but it's wonderfully strengthening. Bath milks made with juniper oil are energising but also make you feel pleasantly tired, so they are ideal for using at night to support regeneration after a strenuous day at work. This oil is most effective when used in an oil dispersion bath (see page 121).

Good for your soul

A thousand things that all need to get done at once, trying not to forget anything or lose your focus – that's what a stress type's day looks like. Of course it's a significant contributing factor in high blood pressure, which makes it all the more important for you to find ways of coming to peace without adding to your already jam-packed appointment calendar.

There are many relaxation methods you may find useful: Autogenic Training, Focusing, or Jacobson's progressive muscle relaxation, to name just a few.

One method that has proven especially effective for high blood pressure is meditation. It does not require special clothing or the ability to sit in the lotus position. You can meditate at home as easily as during a break at the office. You can even fit in five minutes of meditation on the bus or train.

Keep your kidneys warm!

Keep the kidney area of your back (roughly waist level) warm with a sleeveless angora undershirt. It protects this sensitive, easily chilled area without adding bulk. It's especially important to pay attention to your kidneys because they are the key organs in blood pressure regulation.

Learn to meditate

In a meditation course, you'll learn what to do when your thoughts wander too much during meditation. Courses are often centred on a 'day of mindfulness' when you spend about eight hours in silence. In the evening, the group gets together to share experiences. Most courses meet once a week for eight weeks, but two-or-three-day intensive seminars are also available.

Neurological studies have shown that the whole body comes to rest in meditation, just as it does during sleep, even though you are wide awake. The heartbeat becomes slower and more regular, breathing becomes deeper, and the sympathetic nervous system (which is not subject to conscious control and is co-responsible for blood pressure) is downregulated.

Mindfulness meditation

There are many types of meditation drawn from Oriental and Christian traditions, from Zen to silent meditation, meditative dance to Transcendental Meditation. Mindfulness meditation is the easiest to master, and it's completely ideology-free. It was developed about 30 years ago by the molecular biologist Dr Jon Kabat-Zinn and is being implemented today in over 240 hospitals and health centres in the US. Mindfulness means directing your attention to the present moment instead of dwelling on the past or future. Perceiving the here and now without judging it or wanting to change it is the point of mindfulness meditation. The best way to master it is by taking a course, but if that's not possible, you can use a CD.

☞ Make sure you have half an hour without interruptions – and be consistent about it! Turn on the answering machine and turn off your mobile phone, TV, and radio. If there is noise you can't turn off, such as the sound of traffic or construction, ignore it as best you can. Also make sure that the room is comfortably warm, and then get started.

☞ Lie down or sit in a relaxed position and close your eyes. Pay attention to nothing other than your breath. Feel it spreading out inside you and then flowing out again, feel your ribcage rising and falling and your stomach gurgling or whatever else you perceive at the moment.

☞ And now the most important thing – just perceive without evaluating anything. If you feel pressure or pain somewhere, don't get annoyed or anxious and don't attempt to ignore or suppress the pain. Simply register what you perceive. Don't take any of it too seriously, but don't disregard anything, either.

☞ After 20–30 minutes, open your eyes again. You should feel calmer than before, and pleasantly refreshed.

☞ If you meditate every day, you should soon notice a significant drop in your blood pressure.

Being mindful wherever you are

You can practise mindfulness at any time – whether you're brushing your teeth, taking a shower, ironing, vacuuming, chopping vegetables, going for a walk, or sorting files. In every situation in life, there is something to be aware of – it's just a question of being alert to it. If you're cutting vegetables, for example, what does the handle of the knife feel like, or the surface of the carrot? What does it look like when the dirt goes down the drain? What do your fingertips feel as they skin an onion? What do you smell at that moment? Mindfulness exercises such as these are easy to incorporate into your daily life.

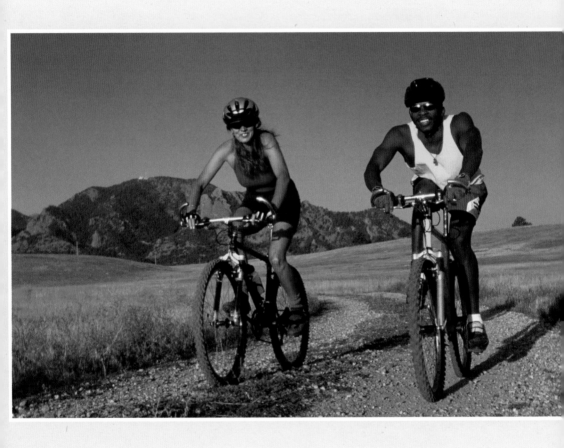

The Programme for Abdominal Types

Do you like to eat well and tend to put on weight? Are you calmness personified and slow to get moving? Do you prefer to be comfortable? Is exercise definitely not one of your major passions? Then you're an abdominal type, and you're on the right track with this programme. It's designed to get you out of your comfy chair for a bit and to expose you to new enjoyment of your surroundings and the natural world. You'll find it will also help you lighten up a bit.

Successful treatments

On pages 53 and 54 you read about the struggles of Henry J. and Ricarda S. and especially about how hopeless Ricarda's situation seemed.

Her example, however, shows how much type-specific high blood pressure therapy can accomplish with an appropriate approach.

Case study 3: Henry J.

When Henry J. (see page 53) comes to the clinic for in-patient treatment, the doctors and therapists help him work out an individualised treatment that he can easily continue at home.

Every day begins with a refreshing rosemary/sea salt scrub (see page 121). A new dietary plan is designed to help him lose weight. Henry had been accustomed to eating his main meal at night – a habit that encourages deposition of abdominal fat – so his big meal is moved to midday and emphasises vegetarian entrées. Twice a week Henry has a fruit juice day. Over the course of the day, he drinks 4 litres (3 ½ quarts) of diluted fruit juices (his choice of either refreshing citrus juices or a mixture of different fruits). Juice fasting fosters alertness and activates body and soul. Between 'meals' he drinks detox teas (see box on the next page). If he can't get through the day without solid food, a rice dish can be added to the juice or tea, and if two juice days per week prove to be too much, one will also do. As a general rule, it's suggested that he drink a lot: all kinds of herb teas and juices, with as much variety as possible. He has a choice of one of these beverages or a piece of fresh fruit for his between-meal 'snacks'.

Henry goes for an easy half-hour walk twice a day, walking until he begins to sweat. Initially, it's not easy for him, but when he gets back from his little excursions he notices how much better he feels. Three times a week he takes a rosemary oil dispersion bath (see page 121) and does curative eurythmy (see page 161) and speech formation. To support the therapeutic process, Henry takes anthroposophical medications (see page 147) such as Ferrum sidereum D20. After ten days, his blood pressure has normalised and the scales show that he has lost 4 kilos (½ stone). The only antihypertensive drug he still needs is an ACE inhibitor (see page 144). Henry goes home feeling generally stronger, and his success in the hospital encourages him to stick to his new diet and daily exercise. He plans to get a dog, which will be a good incentive to get out in the fresh air regardless of the weather.

Detox teas

Certain herbal teas that stimulate the metabolism encourage rapid elimination of waste products. A time-tested mixture for this purpose includes equal proportions of calendula flowers; leaves of stinging nettle, blackberry, and birch; plus yarrow and lemon balm. Drink 1–3 cups daily.

Case study 4: Ricarda S.

When Ricarda (see page 54) comes to the clinic, she tips the scales at 50 kilos (7 ½ stone) over her ideal weight. She is withdrawn and despondent. To stimulate and refresh her, she is prescribed a daily sponge bath with lemon and sea salt each morning in an addition to rosemary oil dispersion baths three times a week (see page 121) and rhythmic massage (see page 163). She does curative eurythmy and speech formation every day (see page 161). She is initially skeptical and doesn't know what to make of these strange therapies, but then she begins to experience herself in a totally new way through the curative eurythmy gestures and especially in speech formation. She begins to feel more aware of her body and to perceive herself better. She notices how she always tended to work everything out on her own, and allowed not feeling well to render her voiceless, hiding within herself. Now she experiences how good it feels to say something out loud. She hears the sounds of the syllables and takes pleasure in reciting beautiful poems. Initially, she just mumbles the words, but the therapist encourages her to speak each syllable loudly and articulate clearly. Gradually, she finds her voice again. She takes St. John's wort drops (Hypericum D3, see page 160) for depression, along with homeopathically diluted gold. Her mood improves after only a few days. She even has the courage to make an appointment for therapy with

105

a psychologist. She wants to get rid of what is tormenting her and is now willing to accept help from outside. She also learns to say no on occasion and terminates friendships that are not good for her. Anthroposophical medications such as Ferrum sidereum D20, Cardiodoron, and a poultice of Aurum/Lavandula comp. (see page 156) over the heart support her in this process. Gradually, a sensitive woman who can finally recognise her own positive qualities is revealed.

To treat her high blood sugar, the doctor switches her from tablets to insulin injections, along with a crash course in nutrition. Ricarda checks her blood sugar three times a day and calculates her insulin dose accordingly. She shifts her diet to lots of vegetables, fruit, lean meat, fish, and wholegrain products. She loses no weight during her stay at the clinic but is already 2 kilos (4 lb) lighter after a week at home. Within the next two months, she loses 14 kilos (2 stone) more, and her blood pressure slowly settles down to normal levels. Of her conventional medications, Ricarda continues to take only a low dose of an ACE inhibitor. She gradually begins to go outside again – initially just for a walk around the block, but in the following weeks she ventures farther from home in ever-expanding circles, gradually reclaiming her extended living space. Life has her back again – and she has her life back.

Plump but healthy

Being overweight isn't always entirely negative. If you're pleasingly plump but mobile and active, that's fine. People of this type have a thick layer of subcutaneous fat rather than a lot of abdominal fat. There's no reason to worry about excess weight if it's not accompanied by diabetes, high triglyceride levels, and low blood levels of HDL cholesterol. Most individuals like this need their ample natural padding in order to stay healthy and active.

Different types of depression

There are three distinctly different types of depression:

☞ Your thoughts run in circles; you never come to rest or find a way out, but go round and round as if caught on a treadmill. This type of depression is especially common in stress types.

☞ You feel paralysed. Daily chores such as getting up, getting dressed, and going shopping feel like almost insurmountable obstacles. The future is a complete fog. Despondency and loss of perspective predominate, and any sense of life's meaning is long since lost. This form of depression most frequently affects abdominal types.

☞ You no longer perceive beauty; sensory perception fades, and with it your enthusiasm. Bleakness and a feeling of separation from your personal and social environment predominate. Having conversations or communicating in other ways becomes almost impossible. It's as if a curtain has been drawn between you and your surroundings. This type of depression frequently affects chaos types and is often associated with burn-out.

Developing a mindful lifestyle

Abdominal types usually need some incentive to become truly active, so we've compiled a wide variety of options for you. They're fun, you'll see! And the best thing about them is that your blood pressure will go down.

Getting off to a good start

Many abdominal types like to sleep late and have a hard time getting out of bed. Here are some tricks that will make getting up a quicker and happier process:

☞ Set your alarm clock early enough to allow adequate time for getting dressed and washed and having a bit of breakfast.

☞ Allow yourself an extra ten minutes in bed, but sit up and review your plans for the day. What's on your calendar? What do you want to accomplish today? (Don't anticipate getting more done than you can actually manage!)

☞ Then stand up and do five minutes of morning exercises – a few stretches are enough.

☞ If you have a garden and it's a warm time of year, you can go outside barefoot (even if it's raining) instead of doing those morning exercises. Take a few deep breaths and become aware of what you are seeing, hearing, and smelling. Then dry your feet vigorously but quickly, and hustle back inside for a warm shower!

☞ Put on your favourite music and dance briskly for a few minutes.

☞ Indulge in a small but nutritious breakfast – for example, warm oatmeal with fresh or dried fruit, or muesli with yogurt.

☞ Instead of rushing off to work half-asleep, follow this morning routine to get yourself active before breakfast.

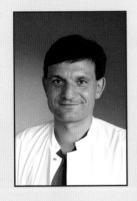

My personal tip

Every day at the same time!

The exercise that follows was developed by Rudolf Steiner, the founder of anthroposophy. It offers you, as an abdominal type, a way to train your will. Initially, the exercise sounds a bit ridiculous, but if you do it consistently for several weeks, you'll notice that you're becoming more assertive and strong-minded. The exercise consists simply of deciding on a specific time and then doing something you've also specified – not necessarily something useful or meaningful! – at that time every day. For example, you could move an ornament from left to right on a shelf and move it back in the opposite direction the next day, or you could make a picture hang crooked on one day and straighten it the next – whatever occurs to you. It's essential to repeat the action every day at the same time, to make no changes to the routine, and to blithely disregard the fact that the action is essentially nonsense. The experience of accomplishing your intention is all that counts.

Stimulate your senses

As an abdominal type, you need strong sensory stimulation in order to feel alert and ready for action, and it's easiest to get that stimulation outdoors. Take every opportunity to open up your senses consciously, whether it's on a shopping trip or on your way to work: what colour is the sky today? How do the trees look? What sounds do you hear; what can you smell?

Is it windy or calm? What does the surface you're walking on feel like? Lift your face to the raindrops and let a few fall into your mouth – how does the water taste? Do these sensory exercises every time you have an errand to run. Walk or cycle to work if at all possible. If you take public transport, get out one stop before your destination and walk the rest of the way. Or park your car where you'll still have a ten-minute walk. These are easy ways to create opportunities for sensory exercises so you'll begin your working day alert and in a good mood.

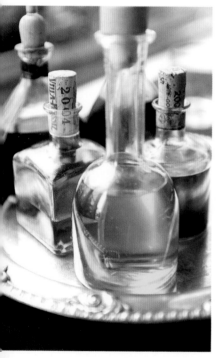

High quality, cold-pressed vegetable oils are a must-have in every well-stocked kitchen.

Type-appropriate nutrition

Good food typically plays a big role in the life of abdominal types, and we certainly don't want to spoil your enjoyment of it. Quite the contrary! We want to show you how you can eat tasty food, feel full, and still lose weight if you need to.

Low-fat doesn't mean no-fat

If you're overweight, you should eat fat sparingly, but it's important to choose the right kinds of fat:

☞ Cold-pressed olive or canola oil is ideal for sauces and salads.

☞ Fatty deep-sea fish (mackerel, herring, salmon) contain valuable omega-3 fatty acids that prevent inflammation in the arteries and lower triglyceride levels (see page 44) as well as blood pressure. Milder fish from shallow ocean waters and freshwater fish are also rich in these valuable oils.

☞ Peanut and sesame oils are the best ones for frying. Both of them can be used for high heat cooking without burning and releasing hazardous substances.

☞ Avoid coconut and palm oils along with hydrogenated fats (including margarine) and convenience foods that contain them (like commercial baked goods and instant sauces and soups).

☞ You don't need to give up hearty home cooking such as roast pork, French fries, and potato salad completely – after all, we want you to continue to enjoy your food. The most important point is to use high-quality ingredients and choose healthy cooking methods.

☞ You can make 'fries' or 'chips' from fresh potatoes by cooking them in a lightly oiled pan, which uses very little fat.

☞ Trim the fat from your bacon or roast, leaving only a thin layer or none at all.

☞ When you make potato salad, skip the mayonnaise and season it with onions, herbs, broth, mustard, and pickled gherkins.

Lose weight without feeling hungry

Here's a simple trick for losing weight without feeling hungry: choose a high-protein diet. The body has places to deposit sugar and fat, which can then serve as instantly available energy sources. Protein, however, is processed immediately, never stored, and always metabolically active. High-protein foods include lean meat (preferably organic), skinless poultry, fish, milk and dairy products, legumes, tofu, and nuts (including almonds).

111

The glycemic index

All carbohydrates are digested with the help of proteins in the intestines, where they are broken down into simple sugars that are then absorbed into the bloodstream, raising blood sugar levels and triggering insulin secretion. How quickly that happens depends on how the carbohydrates in foods are 'packaged'. With dextrose, soft drinks, or sweets, which all have a high glycemic index or 'GI', it happens very swiftly, but if the carbohydrates are combined with plenty of fibre, it takes a relatively long time for them to be broken down into simple sugars in the small intestine, and blood sugar levels rise slowly. In other words, these foods have a low GI. Fat also slows carbohydrate absorption by delaying the emptying of the stomach. That's why your blood sugar rises only slowly after you eat a piece of chocolate or a scoop of ice cream. In addition to sugars, starches – such as those in mashed potatoes, for example – are also processed quickly and cause rapid increases in blood sugar. Insulin is secreted in sudden, excessive bursts so the cells can process the sugar. These excessive insulin responses are just as harmful as constantly elevated insulin levels. Both decrease cellular sensitivity to insulin, thus promoting insulin resistance and type 2 diabetes. This means you should make a point of eating as many low glycemic index foods as possible, such as:

☞ Apples, apricots, grapefruit, oranges, tangerines, cherries, peaches, blueberries, raspberries.

☞ Aubergine (eggplant), all salad greens, broccoli and all other cruciferous vegetables, chicory, green beans, cucumbers, legumes, chard, peppers, mushrooms, radishes, celery, soya beans, spinach, tomatoes, courgette (zucchini), onions.

☞ Milk and milk products such as yogurt, quark, buttermilk, soured milk, cheeses.

☞ Whole grains such as bulgur, buckwheat, quinoa, rolled oats, millet; whole-grain bread and muesli; whole wheat noodles; brown rice; semolina and noodles made from durum wheat.

Fruits for a sweet tooth

Do you love desserts? Try tropical fruits instead of chocolate mousse. For example, lemon sorbet is very tasty but not at all fattening. If citrus is too tart for your taste, try pomegranates, kumquats, ground cherries, passion fruit, mango, or papaya for a delicious change.

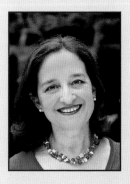

My personal tip

Try oats

If you're at risk of diabetes or already have diabetes or metabolic syndrome, you should eat oats once or twice a week. Even a small quantity of oats is very filling, and oats can reduce the need for insulin and improve cellular insulin resistance. There are many different ways to prepare oats – give them a sweet spin with fresh or dried fruit or savoury with broth and herbs. If you use different seasonings each time, your porridge will always taste new and different! (see also pages 90-91)

As well as eating plenty of low GI foods, you should avoid high GI foods whenever possible. These include:

☞   Potato dishes such as chips and fries, potato croquettes, instant mashed potatoes.

☞   Cornflakes and all other commercial sweetened cereals; cornstarch, white rice, rice cakes.

113

☞ White flour products such as bagels, rolls, croissants, cookies, biscuits, waffles, muffins.

☞ Sodas and colas (with the exception of diet products).

☞ Commercial fruit juices, white and brown sugar, honey, maple syrup, fructose, maltose, dextrose, and jams and preserves made with sugar.

Season without salt

If you're a 'salt sensitive' individual (see page 45) whose blood pressure drops only when you consume less salt, you should:

☞ Ban salt-shakers, liquid seasonings, and instant broths from your kitchen and dining room and prepare all your foods with fresh or dried herbs.

☞ Replace salt with exotic spices that have strong flavours of their own, such as chilli, paprika, garlic, cloves, nutmeg, cumin, ginger, black pepper, and cardamom.

☞ Season salads simply with balsamic vinegar and a few drops of good olive oil instead of a salty dressing.

☞ Avoid frozen foods and convenience foods, which are always salted. At the bakery counter, ask about reduced-salt breads.

☞ Replace sodium and chlorine-laden mineral water with low-sodium brands, or just drink tap water.

☞ Avoid cured meats and marinated fish whenever possible.

☞ Instead of chips, peanut snacks, pretzel sticks, or salted nuts, eat fruit salad while you're watching television.

Keep it crunchy!

As an abdominal type, you need crunchy food, because the more you have to chew, the more consciously you eat. If you don't like your vegetables raw, blanch them for a minute or two in salted water so they're slightly softened but still have some bite. Vegetables that respond well to this treatment include carrots, kohlrabi, cauliflower, broccoli, white and red cabbage, sweet peppers, beetroot, celery, and courgettes.

Fruit and vegetables: five a day

We're sure you've heard this recommendation before: you should eat five servings of vegetables or fruit every day; a total of 600–700 g (just over 1 lb). They provide important vitamins, minerals, and trace elements that your body needs to carry out its metabolic processes. Some even help capture free radicals, which are harmful substances that can promote deposits in the blood vessels – an especially undesirable situation if you have high blood pressure. Fruits and vegetables contain important antioxidants that prevent the inflammation response that occurs when free radicals attack the sensitive inner walls of blood vessels. In addition, yellow, red, and green vegetables contain natural plant protectants (such as polyphenols) that promote the body's own defences and stimulate fat metabolism, which is especially good for your heart and circulation. It's easy to get in five servings over the course of the day. At breakfast, mix fruit into yoghurt or muesli or make yourself a fruit salad. Sometime between breakfast and lunch, drink a glass of fruit or vegetable juice (diluted with water, if need be). At lunch, have vegetables or a big salad as either a side dish or main dish. At your evening meal, you can enjoy a helping of salad, crudités, or

115

another portion of fruit. And by the way, you can drink beetroot juice as often as you like: it lowers blood pressure (see page 95).

Steer clear of snacks

As an abdominal type who enjoys eating, you're especially susceptible to snacking between meals, but you're better off sticking to three main meals a day. Here are some tricks that will help you avoid feeling ravenous between meals.

☞ An hour before eating lunch or dinner, have a piece of fruit (preferably an apple). Apples contain valuable minerals and vitamins and will help you feel full. They even lower your blood pressure!

☞ Instead of reaching for a snack, have something to drink – a cup of chai, for example, which is an Indian spiced tea containing ginger, cardamom, black pepper, cloves, cinnamon, and anise. Tea shops carry many different variations. Boil the spice mixture for 10–20 minutes, then add warm milk and honey. These aromatic teas are warming and stimulate the metabolism. If you're trying to lose weight, skip the milk and use less honey.

Fasting and detoxing

One fast day per week or month can work wonders if you make a habit of it. Fasting gives your body a chance to emphasise the breakdown aspect of metabolism. No deposition takes place; you're simply using up what's already there (especially fat, which is exactly what you want to achieve). The body benefits the most from fasting at regular, rhythmic intervals, which allows it to 'tune in' to the process

After a fast, you'll notice that you feel wonderfully light and invigorated. You can feel how good it is for your body to not have to be involved in digestion for a whole day. And fasting does not mean that you can't eat anything. Your meals should be small, very light, and include plenty to drink, for example:

For a rice-and-fruit or rice-and-juice day: three times a day, eat 50 g (⅓ cup) of cooked brown rice combined with 900g (2 lb) fruit or 1–2 litres (8 cups) of fruit juice. Rice is a diuretic, so it drives accumulated fluids out of the body. The fruits or juices ensure that you get enough vitamins. They also get your metabolism going and have a refreshing effect.

For a fruit day: eat 1–2 kilos (3–4 lb) of fruits of various types, either fresh or steamed. (Don't add sugar!) Juicy varieties such as melons, strawberries, raspberries, apples, pears, oranges, and grapefruits are best. To drink, you can have tea, broth, or an assortment of diluted juices.

Eat your evening meal earlier

Eat as little as possible at night and nothing at all after 7 pm. Or cancel dinner entirely once a week. Hearty evening meals sit heavy on your stomach at night and make you sluggish well into the next day. A better choice is to have your main meal in the middle of the day, preferably complete with an appetizer, an entrée, and a dessert. If your stomach growls in the evening, pacify it with an apple.

Exercise and physical activity

For abdominal types, physical activity is the single most important way to get rid of abdominal fat. It only begins to melt away when you really break a sweat, which is a sign that your body is burning its fat reserves. But physical activity is good for your well-being in general. It not only energises you, it increases your enjoyment of life – assuming that you actually do enjoy the movement, that is! Physical activity should not feel like a burden or an

117

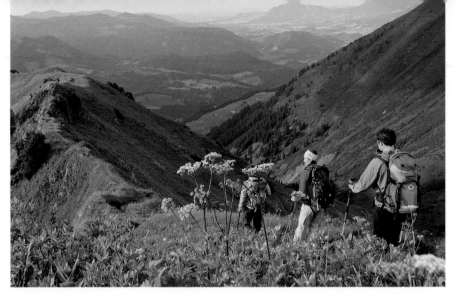

Nature walks are ideal for abdominal types. Outdoor exercise lowers blood pressure and opens your senses to wind, clouds, sunlight, and quiet reflection.

obligation you impose on yourself only for the sake of your health. You need to enjoy it and feel that you're benefiting from it, so choose an activity that you really like and do it every day, if at all possible.

As a general rule, all endurance sports are excellent for abdominal types: hiking, swimming, cross-country skiing, jogging, Nordic walking, cycling, dancing, gymnastics. But even going for a walk is good, if you step out freely and don't just stroll along. Less suitable – but still better than nothing – are horseback riding, downhill skiing, bowling, tennis, football, and handball.

Games that are not too physically challenging are also good: volleyball, table tennis, billiards or snooker, golf.

If you like, you can also build up you strength and endurance at a fitness centre, but don't force yourself to go – you can meet your goals without a gym membership.

You may find outdoor exercise easier if you combine it with a meaningful volunteer activity: take the neighbourhood kids along on a hike, take special-needs adults for a walk, or take part in a clean-up day in a local forest or greenbelt. If you're good at identifying bird songs, invite friends and neighbors to go bird-watching. (In big cities, major cemeteries are good places for this!)

Good for your body

To wake up in the morning, abdominal types need stimulation from outside. That's why rub-downs with sea salt and either rosemary or lemon (see page 121) are so pleasant for you. You'll feel your energy increase and face the day feeling wonderfully refreshed.

Massages and saunas

As an abdominal type, you should indulge in a massage now and then. The pressure should be neither too light nor too hard – just enough for good body awareness, especially on your back, arms, and legs. Many abdominal types simply blank out these body parts as if they didn't exist. Adequate sensation is essential, however, especially in your legs – after all, they allow you to walk – so more vigorous massaging, which enlivens metabolism, is appropriate on your calves and thighs. If your hands and feet tend to get cold and go numb, a massage can 'wake them up' again. So can a session in the sauna. It's best not to start off with a Finnish-style sauna at 95 °C (203 °F). Instead, choose a sweat lodge or a wellness sauna at 65–80 °C (140–180 °F). After your session, take a quick lukewarm shower and then hop into the ice-cold plunge pool. In winter, going outside and running naked through the snow serves the same purpose: the sensation of cold after heat stimulates and activates your entire body. Your skin tingles and comes alive. The Scandinavian custom of lightly whipping the whole body with birch twigs during or right after a sauna session also gives an overall sensation of well-being. It shouldn't hurt, but you should definitely be able to feel it as it revs up your circulation and makes your skin nicely rosy.

How exercise helps

Endurance sports have a direct effect on blood pressure. At rest, only 3–5% of the capillaries (see page 16) are open, but with exertion the number of open capillaries increases by 30–50 times and their total surface area by about 100 times. This decreases resistance to the flow of blood the heart pumps out into the body, causing your blood pressure to drop.

Hot-and-cold showers

To take a hot-and-cold shower, first shower normally, then briefly turn the spray to hot until you get really warm. Then unscrew the shower head so the water comes out of the tube in a thick stream and turn the tap to cold – as cold as it will get, not just lukewarm. Run this stream quickly over your whole body, beginning with the outside of your right calf, up the hip, and down the inside. Repeat on the left leg. Then do the outside and inside of your arms, and finally move in a clockwise circle over your abdomen and around your chest. Finish with a quick splash on your face – use your hands or aim the stream right at your face – and you're done.

Another option is to leave the shower head on and guide the spray over your body, moving somewhat faster and alternating between hot and cold three times. Or rub your whole body down with an exfoliating bath mitt or a loofah, either during your shower or afterward, before applying a body lotion. Birch oil is also good for skin care: extract of young birch leaves can help flush excess water and metabolic waste out of the body. All of these stimulating options are wonderfully refreshing and raise your spirits.

Sea salt: a good way to start the day

Coarse sea salt contains many minerals and trace elements, and its granular texture makes it a good exfoliant. Try it during your morning shower: dribble a bit of rosemary or lemon bath milk on to an exfoliating bath mitt and wring it out lightly, then sprinkle on some salt and scrub your entire body with it. Then rinse the salt off with lukewarm water and finish – if you like – with a cold splash. You'll enjoy how your skin feels when your circulation is revved up.

Oil dispersion baths

Oil doesn't dissolve in water, so when you use an ordinary oil-based bath product, the droplets inevitably end up floating on the surface within a very short time. That's not the case with an oil dispersion bath (Jungebad). Instead, the oil is very finely distributed throughout the entire volume of water, and the combination remains stable for days. If you left the water standing in the tub, it would take a week for the oil droplets to rise slowly to the surface. This is possible with the help of a special device, invented in 1937 by medical balneotherapist Werner Junge, that remains very popular with physical therapists even today The device is also easy to use at home.

For an oil dispersion bath, use only the finest pure olive oil combined with etheric oils of medicinal herbs to suit your needs: rosemary is enlivening, lavender calming, rose protects, St. John's wort is warming and strengthens the nerves, monkshood eases pain. There are roughly 70 different kinds of oils that can be used as needed.

121

Be realistic

We're sure you're familiar with this scenario: you have great plans that you don't accomplish, and at the end of the day you're left moaning, 'Oh, if only I could actually get everything done!' A better approach is to take on only as much as you can actually accomplish and gradually increase your self-imposed quota. Being able to look back on the day with a sense of accomplishment will allow you to plan the next day with more motivation and a pleasant sense of anticipation.

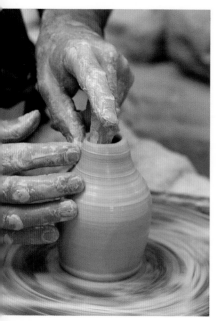

Throwing pots is relaxing... and it awakens your creativity.

Good for your soul

If you tend to be most comfortable within your own four walls, try to cultivate new interests to counteract the tendency to take it easy.

☞ Attend local cultural events instead of simply watching TV or listening to the radio.

☞ Check out the course listings at your local adult education center. There's bound to be something there to suit your interests.

☞ Learn to play an instrument.

☞ Sign up for an art course or learn a craft: drawing, painting, pottery, handicrafts, felting, embroidery, sewing, rug hooking, weaving, or knitting. Many florists also offer courses in flower arranging or ikebana.

122

☞   During any creative activity, you'll feel yourself getting warm. That's because your body is breaking down the energy reserves you've built up from your food. This happens not only during athletic activity but whenever you do anything actively and deliberately, because your will's intention can express itself only when your brain burns sugar and oxygen.

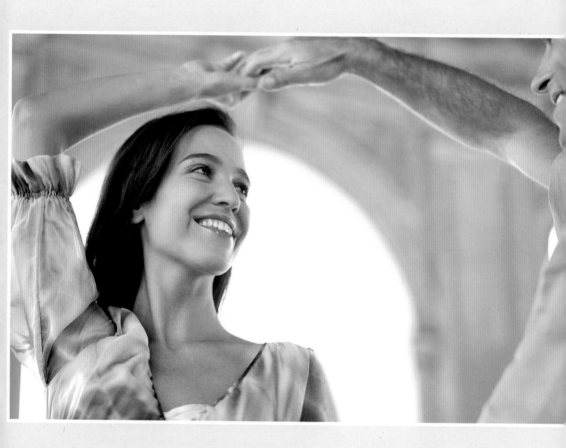

The Programme for Chaos Types

Both stress and abdominal types are subject to one-sidedness that can become unhealthy, but what chaos types lack is the harmony in the middle. Think of a seesaw, which is only in balance when both ends are up in the air. Chaos types can't sustain this balance and sometimes tend toward the stress type, sometimes toward the abdominal type. Bringing rhythm into the structure of their daily life gently corrects these imbalances. The basic health-promoting tips in this section are relevant for anyone of any age or in any situation in life, and for men as well as women.

Successful treatments

Do you remember our two examples of chaos types, Manuela S. and Joseph B? In spite of prescription drugs, they were unable to get their blood pressure under control. Healing changes could only begin after doctors recognised the underlying causes of their severe blood pressure fluctuations.

Case study 5: Manuela S.

Manuela S. (see page 56) comes to the clinic reluctantly, bringing her infant with her. Her worrying physical condition (she is seriously underweight) makes the stay in hospital necessary. Everything is in good hands at home: her husband and sister are managing the household and taking care of the other two children. The first instruction she gets from the doctor is: wean that baby! Her problems began when she was pregnant and have grown even worse while breastfeeding, and nothing will change as long as Manuela is so intensely involved with her infant. Her own restlessness is transmitted directly to the baby, so neither of them gets any rest during the day. Manuela needs to be able to reconnect with herself.

Actually, she would be a classic case for conventional medical treatment with a beta blocker and an antidepressant, but would that help her find her centre? No. So the doctors try a different approach, reaching deep into their treasure chest of anthroposophical medicines (see page 147). Manuela receives Stibium D6 intravenously three times a day, an intravenous injection of Aurum D10 each morning, Hyoscyamus D6 drops three times a day, Bryophyllum mother tincture (drops) three times a day, and Galenit D4 (powder) three times a day. All of this is designed to help quiet her nerves, slow her heartbeat, and promote relaxation. The attempt is initially not very successful. In the first week, the weaning causes breast engorgement, which makes everything else worse. Manuela has no appetite and is almost unable to eat. The doctors switch her from Hyoscyamus D6 to Hyoscyamus D3/Argentum D8, which can be administered subcutaneously and is well tolerated even if the patient is nauseous.

But Manuela still feels helpless. Free-form therapeutic painting (see page 162) makes her very agitated, so the therapist recommends rhythmical form-drawing, a more structured therapy that calms Manuela's breathing and allows her to come to peace inwardly. Curative eurythmy and rhythmic massage (see page 161 and 163) and whole-body rubs with lavender oil do even more good. Her blood pressure normalises and her appetite returns. Her underlying mood of anxiety and her psychological chaos persists, however, so the doctors decide to prescribe an antidepressant (citalopram). Manuela is homesick for her family, so her treatment is continued on an out-patient basis. Together with her doctors, she designs a schedule that allows her to cope effectively with her familiar daily routine, inserting repeated breaks. Two weeks later, her situation has improved significantly. Manuela is working with a psychotherapist to process her anxieties and plans to stop taking the antidepressant as soon as possible. Her blood pressure has already settled down to normal levels.

Rhythm supports life

The life of the body depends on rhythmical functions. Specific rhythms underlie not only breathing, digestion, and the beating of the heart, but also all metabolic processes and the production of neurotransmitters. Illness results when natural rhythms are consistently ignored. (Many digestive disorders, for example, can be traced back to irregular eating habits.) That's why many medical approaches to healing aim to stimulate and restore the body's rhythmical regulatory processes.

Case study 6: Joseph B.

When Joseph B (see page 57) is admitted to the hospital to learn how to normalise his blood pressure, he has a concert scheduled for the following weekend. Cancelling this engagement is extremely difficult for him because he has always made a point of doing everything he agrees to do. But he has promised to do something for himself, and the situation demands that he take that promise seriously. He finally reschedules the concert.

Joseph has been taking a number of medications, and his doctors start by taking him off beta blockers (see page 145). He continues to take a lower dose of the ACE inhibitor (see page 144). In addition, the doctors prescribe some anthroposophical medications (see page 147).

Joseph is prescribed Cardiodoron, Cuprum metallicum praeparatum D8 for insomnia, Aurum D10 at noon, and a compress of Aurum and Lavandula comp. (see page 156) applied over the heart in the morning upon waking and at night before going to sleep. The purpose of the compresses is to help him face the day and night more calmly and to shape and experience these transitions consciously. In the morning, he uses the fifteen minutes while the compress is applied to his chest to preview the day: what's on my schedule today? What can I plan to get done? What do I need to pay special attention to? In the evening, he reviews the events of the day: what happened today? How do I feel now? What went well? What could have been done better?

24-hour monitoring indicates in spite of his newly structured daily routine, Joseph's blood pressure shoots up whenever emotions come to the surface – for example, when he admits to uncertainties or expresses and processes feelings he used to suppress. Curative eurythmy and rhythmical massage are helpful but cannot completely restore the balance.

After a week in the hospital, Joseph is eager to go home, and the doctors agree, with the following stipulations. He must sit down to a hot meal once a day, and eat it calmly and with enjoyment. He will pay attention to eating enough bitter-tasting foods (see box opposite); his diet is to be low in fat and meat but otherwise aromatic and varied. For half an hour every day, he will take a fast walk or get some other form of enjoyable exercise. He will work out a schedule for the year with his wife, arranging all of his engagements to allow him to spend time at home in between.

After following these recommendations conscientiously for a year, Joseph's blood pressure has normalised completely. His daily routine is no longer dominated by his concert schedule, and overall his life has become calmer and more satisfying.

Bitter foods

Bitter-tasting foods are both stimulating and strengthening. Bitter greens (such as chicory, radicchio, rocket, and endive in salads) and seasonings (such as orange, lemon, or lime zest in salads or sauces) produce a pleasant sensation of well-being in the body yet without making you feel tired – just right for restoring balance in a chaos type.

Developing a mindful lifestyle

Losing rhythm and flexibility of response generally has little to do with pre-disposition and constitution, and more to do with lifestyle factors, especially lack of rhythm in daily life. Restoring this rhythm is essential for chaos types but is also helpful for stress and abdominal types as well – or indeed, for anyone. Rhythm is life-supporting and energising and eases the burden of stress, and not just for people with high blood pressure. Leading a rhythmical life fundamentally strengthens the body and prevents all sorts of diseases, which usually reflect the fact that the body has got out of rhythm and become pathologically one-sided. The basic idea is very simple: it's enough to choose one thing to do every day at the same time: meals, waking up or going to sleep, a coffee break, a walk, or morning exercise. Whatever you choose, it should fit with your personal lifestyle and you should do it every day at approximately the same time. Why? Because everything you do at rhythmical intervals becomes habitual, so it gets a little easier each

129

time. Even on the psychological level, rhythm inserts moments of calm into a hectic schedule. For that reason alone, it is essential for modern life. Take a look at our lifestyle recommendations for stress types (see page 99–100) – tips on how to get out of the fast lane and enjoy a slower and more pleasant life. These suggestions also apply to chaos types.

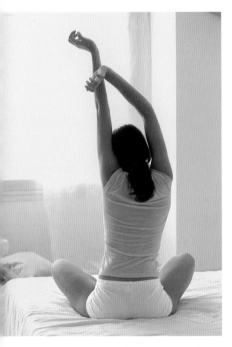

A good stretch when you wake up is very refreshing!

Sleeping soundly

The alternation between sleeping and waking is one of the most important and basic human rhythms. Like inhaling and exhaling, giving and receiving, it is a fundamental rhythm of life, and even today its secret depths have not been fully fathomed. No one can say where we are when we are sleeping. We only know that brain activity is put in stand-by mode when we sleep, and our consciousness takes a break from sending and receiving.

We also know that during sleep, regeneration takes place and many bodily processes are adjusted. Cultivating sound sleep at night is the deciding factor in being alert and 'present'.

Getting a good night's sleep

☞ If possible, go to bed at the same time every night, preferably by 11 pm at the latest. You sleep most deeply between midnight and 3 am; that's when restorative processes are strongest.

☞ Eat little or nothing after 8 pm. Anything you eat then should be light, or you won't be able to sleep well.

☞ Don't channel-surf before going to sleep. Set a limit for yourself: at 10 pm, the TV is turned off, and later programmes get recorded for future viewing.

☞ Make sure that your feet are nice and warm when you get into bed.

☞ Develop a going-to-sleep ritual. Rhythmic repetition is strengthening and balancing. Say a poem, a prayer, or an affirmation so you'll fall asleep thinking good thoughts.

How to feel more rested

Are you a chaos type who complains about not sleeping well and feeling tired all the time? Take a close look at whether you're having trouble *falling asleep* or *waking up*. These imbalances are characteristic of stress and abdominal types, respectively. Here's how to get back in balance:

☞ If you're sleeping badly, try to be as alert and focused as possible during the day. The more presence, consciousness, and alertness you can muster during the day, the more likely you are to feel naturally tired and sleep well at night. If you sense your concentration flagging in the course of the day, take a short break for a few deep breaths out in the fresh air.

☞ Conversely, if you have trouble waking up, go to bed an hour or two before midnight. Consciously plan in a quiet time for your going-to-sleep ritual: listen to your favorite music; take a warm footbath and then rub your feet with lavender oil; read a book or listen to someone else read aloud. After this gentle transition into sleep, you'll sleep more soundly and wake up truly rested and refreshed.

How to wake up

☞ Set the alarm for fifteen minutes earlier than necessary and spend those minutes looking ahead to the day. Before you even get up, plan your day: what would be the best way to divide up your morning, afternoon, and evening? What must you remember? The more you anticipate, the less chaotic your day will be.

☞ Allow plenty of time for showering, getting dressed, and having a leisurely breakfast.

☞ Allow enough time to drive or walk to work without rushing. Time your departure so you get to work a few minutes early.

Organise your day

As you look ahead to the day, think through the events and organise them carefully:

☞ What can I expect to encounter today?

☞ Who will be expecting something of me, and what will those expectations involve?

☞ When and where will my strengths be needed?

This train of thought will free you from chaotic thinking. You'll become calmer – and your blood pressure will drop!

The power of poetry

Even if you haven't recited a poem in a long time, you should do it daily from now on. It can help synchronise heartbeat and respiration and bring a harmonious rhythm into your day.

It's a good idea to spend ten minutes a day reading poetry aloud. Try 'Invictus' by William Ernest Henley to start you off. There's no need to memorise it; reading aloud from a book is fine. Then choose a suitable sample by your favourite poet, and if possible, take a few lessons from a speech-formation therapist (see page 161) so you learn to get the emphasis right. If you practice this recitation regularly over several weeks or months, you'll notice its harmonising effect.

The therapeutic effect of poetry and singing

In the amphitheatres of ancient Greece, recitations of great poets' works often lasted from early morning to late at night. Homer's *Odyssey* alone consists of more than 10,000 lines of hexameter, and the *Iliad* is even longer. The audience relaxed into the recitation; during attentive listening, breathing and pulse rate settle. Consequently, these epic recitations were not just cultural events; they were also valuable for health reasons. The same is true of Gregorian chants, where short notes are held for one heartbeat and each line can be sung in a single breath. Similarly, chanting mantras and Vedic verses normalises heart rate and lowers blood pressure.

Bringing rhythm to your day

Situations that throw the body out of rhythm include prolonged stress, mistrust, anxiety about the future, and uncertainty about your life, and chaos types should avoid these as much as possible. Of course such stressful situations cannot always be avoided, but if you can anticipate them, you can also take deliberate steps to counteract them – for example, by organising your day even more rhythmically. The best rhythm-enhancers are a regular sleeping schedule and morning and evening rituals. Other things that help are:

☞ Reviewing your daily routine: when and where do things tend to get out of hand? Where should you intervene to establish a more structured sequence of events?

☞ Turning on the answering machine if you don't want to be disturbed at work.

☞ Avoiding becoming a slave to electronic media. Check your email or smartphone only at set times instead of being constantly ready to respond.

☞ Hanging a 'Do not disturb' sign on the door to your room.

☞ Cultivating a culture of taking breaks. If you don't succeed immediately, at least take a half-hour break in the middle of the day and go outside for some fresh air.

☞ Making sure that meal times – especially family meals – are kept free of any interruptions.

☞ Reading aloud to your children or partner in the evening.

☞ Arranging to spend one evening each week with friends. Cook together or do something else you enjoy.

☞ Being consistent about making Sunday a day of rest. Do absolutely nothing that has to do with your work. This will give you time to really 'switch off' so by Monday your head will be clear for the new week's assignments.

Try singing!

Singing lowers your blood pressure and invigorates your breathing. Sung tones are produced only when exhaling, so inhaling and exhaling must be coordinated with the melody – i.e., 'rhythmicised' – which has positive effects on blood pressure.

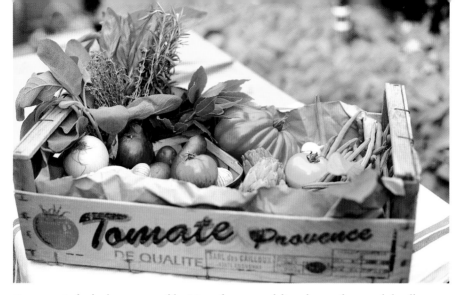

Buy organic food whenever possible. Many farms can deliver boxes of seasonal, locally grown fruit and vegetables.

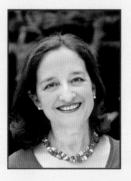

My personal tip

Write it down

For a week, record daily events as they happen – to the quarter hour! Take a close look at which times are already rhythmical and where there are problems. How chaotic is your life? Where can you make adjustments? With practice, you will gradually be able to get your life back on a more structured track.

Type-appropriate nutrition

As a chaos type, the first thing you need to learn is to take time to eat. Don't eat when you're heading out the door or gulp down a sandwich on your way to your next appointment. Plan your day from the start so you have at least enough time for lunch.

☞ At the very least, eat a proper meal once a day – something cooked and tasty; it doesn't need to be a lot. A regular meal brings calmness and structure to your day. It's up to you whether that meal is breakfast, lunch, or supper.

☞ Avoid one-sided eating – don't always eat just salad or just fast food. Aim for a varied diet that offers something different every day.

☞ Pay attention to the quality of your grocery purchases. Buy organic vegetables, eggs, dairy products, and meat.

☞ Go with the seasons and eat only freshly harvested fruit and vegetables from regional organic farms. Eating this way will help you develop a sense for seasonal rhythms.

☞ Stick to the good old rule of the Sunday roast: eating meat once a week is enough, and eating it more than twice a week is not recommended.

☞ 'Fish on Fridays' is also an old Christian custom – although you don't have to limit it to Fridays!

☞ Ideal beverages for you are water, herbal teas, and unsweetened juices, especially beetroot juice.

☞ Depending on whether you tend more toward the stress type or the abdominal type, keep the dietary tips for them in mind, too.

Exercise and physical activity

You guessed it: it doesn't matter how you get your exercise; what's important is to do it regularly – if possible, always on the same day of the week and at the same time. There are many different types of exercise that are valuable for you, especially the ones that emphasise rhythm.

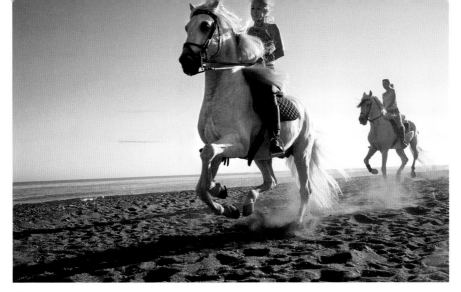

Horse-riding can be a great way to get exercise and fresh air.

☞ Dancing, particularly partner dances such as the waltz, foxtrot, rumba, cha-cha, jive, quickstep, and – the cream of the crop – Argentine tango. When you're dancing, you can leave everything else behind and concentrate completely on your partner and the steps. This is ideal if you have trouble forgetting about your work.

☞ Nordic walking: rhythmical walking with long poles. Hiking is good, too, with its pleasant rhythmical alternation of walking and resting.

☞ Rowing: the ultimate rhythmical exercise. The oar strokes happen at regular intervals but are not identical.

☞ Horseback riding: the horse's rhythmical movements are transmitted to you.

☞ Sailing: exercise plus time to open up to the elements (wind, water, sun) while staying completely focused. Teamwork is an additional plus on larger boats.

☞ Yoga: a perfect opportunity to harmonise bodily rhythms through movements and postures and to achieve both outer and inner balance.

☞ Tai chi and qi gong: thousand-year-old movement patterns that regulate all bodily processes.

Good for your body

You should also look for opportunities for rhythmical alternation when it comes to body care.

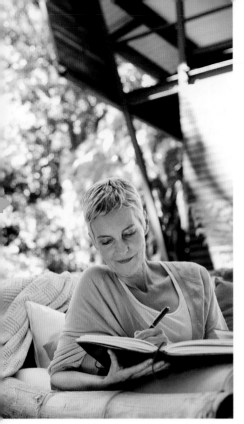

End the day by capturing what you experienced in a few short words.

☞ Use rosemary bath milk during your morning wash to help you really wake up. In the evenings, we recommend a more relaxing lavender bath, but listen to your inner voice: what do you need at the moment? Is it something calming, like lemon balm, valerian, rose, or linden flower, or rather something enlivening, such as mint, lemon, ginger, or camphor? Just experiment!

☞ A whole-body rub with moor lavender oil is especially pleasant in the evening. Begin with your legs, then move on to your arms, and finally massage the oil into your torso with gentle movements in the direction of the heart.

☞ Indulge in a weekly 'relaxation evening' in a sauna or the hamam (Turkish bath with full-body soap wash and massage).

Good for your soul

It's important for chaos types to seek balance on the psychological level, too. This 'centre' is not static; it's a shifting state that you have to repeatedly rediscover. How? By arranging your daily routine as a constant alternation between what you want for yourself and what others need, between self-focus and love for others, autonomy and care-giving. Giving must be balanced by receiving.

☞   Look for tasks or hobbies that make you feel whole inside: get involved in your community or with a social service agency, residential care facility, or youth centre. Plant a garden. Take care of sick neighbours or offer to help with childcare for a single mother. There are countless areas of activity that would welcome your involvement and give you the feeling of being needed and doing something really meaningful.

☞   Along with these activities, take care of yourself, cultivate your hobbies, be there for your family, and create a comfortable home for yourself.

Gain freedom and security

When you find your centre, you can then be receptive to other people, regardless of where you encounter them. By making a habit of anticipating the day (see page 132), you'll develop the presence of mind to draw on the full range of your possibilities. By thinking ahead, you can recognise and acknowledge what is coming toward you. Instead of being at the mercy of events, you face them with freedom and equanimity. Conversely, reviewing the day (see below) helps you meet whatever comes to you with goodwill, appreciation, and tolerance. There's no need to be constantly at odds with destiny; you can simply accept things as they are.

Presence of mind is the middle ground between anticipation and review. It provides security – exactly what a chaos type (or indeed everyone!) needs.

Reviewing the day

When chaos prevails by day, it's important to allow a time in the evening to restore calm and think back on all your stressful experiences. A focussed review of the day needn't take more than ten minutes.

☞   Consider the day's events: what did you experience? Who said what? What did you get excited or upset about?

☞   Acknowledge any feelings of anger or pleasure, but don't judge your responses (or the reasons behind them).

☞   Recognise what happened, accept it; deposit it, and close the door on it.

If you do this review of the day every evening, you will soon stop feeling hopeless about your mistakes. You'll recognise what is good and what needs improvement without feeling guilty about it. Feelings of guilt get us stuck and are almost always unnecessary, since anything that goes wrong usually involves more than one person.

Discover your sources of health

Good health is number one on most people's wish list, but what does being healthy actually mean? The World Health Organization (WHO) defines health as 'a state of complete physical, mental and social well-being'. This utopian definition is something to aspire to, but when do we ever achieve this state? The image painted by Dr Manfred Lütz, a psychiatrist and theologian from Cologne, seems much more realistic: 'A healthy person is someone who can live more or less happily with his or her afflictions'. The art of life, according to Lütz, consists in finding sources of pleasure and ways to enjoy life in spite of handicaps, illness, and suffering. In concrete terms, this means asking yourself: what activities make me feel good? When am I at peace with myself and my surroundings? Which occasions make me feel happy? In short, what personal sources of health help me enjoy life and feel confident?

This concept of 'salutogenesis' (*salus* = health, *genesis* = origin) has become increasingly widespread in recent years. It touches on questions not commonly raised by our modern health-care system, which is primarily oriented toward avoiding disease through preventive programmes, vaccinations, and drugs that seem able to suppress any illness. Of course it makes sense to protect ourselves from disease, but prevention focuses only on illness and pathological factors, whereas salutogenesis concentrates on health and on our own resources. More than just the absence of disease, health means being at peace with ourselves and the world. The body is capable of enduring stress and compensating for it; the soul can spread its wings; we are spiritually active and creative. We oscillate constantly between the two poles of illness and health. They can be experienced only subjectively, through individual, independent activity. That's why there is no such thing as health in general, but only *my* health. It is a means of shaping one's own life as positively as possible.

How can you do that? By accessing your individual physical, spiritual, and psychological sources of health. The physical aspect involves movement, nutrition, and lifestyle; the soul-spiritual aspects entail recognising and accepting your mistakes, maintaining mental flexibility and curiosity, practicing tolerance, listening quietly and respecting the opinions of others, and any and all forms of creativity. In this sense, salutogenesis is a path of daily practice and, like health, must be achieved anew every day – just as your blood pressure adjusts itself repeatedly.

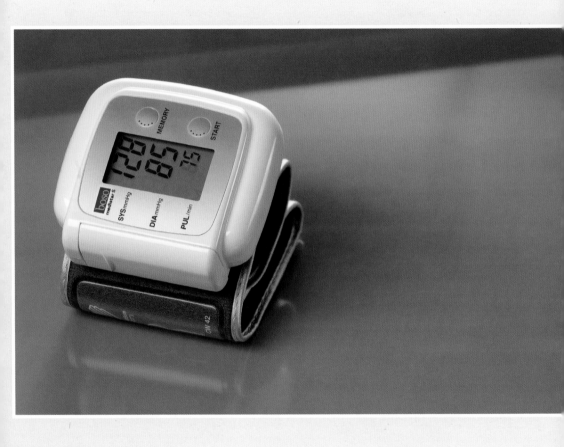

Medical Treatment for Your Type

The right treatment for each type

In consultation with your physician, you may initially decide to attempt to lower your blood pressure by applying the type-specific treatment programme you read about in the preceding chapter, supported by natural medications. The greater your success in improving your overall constitution using these methods, the more effectively you will combat the underlying reasons for high blood pressure; you may even be able to do without any conventional medications at all.

Conventional medication

If your blood pressure remains too high after 3–6 months, you should discuss with your doctor which conventional medication is the best option for you. For decades, diuretics (water pills) and beta blockers were the drugs of choice for treating high blood pressure. They lower blood pressure effectively and have been shown to prevent heart attacks and strokes – but only in a certain percentage of hypertensive patients. What's good for one person may actually be harmful for someone else. Some patients cannot handle these medications at all or complain of significant side effects. For example, stress types treated with diuretics may develop kidney problems, because they tend not to drink a lot of fluids and so the amount of blood in circulation is low. It is always important to keep the patient's individual constitution and life circumstances in mind when selecting hypertensive medications.

In general, all conventional hypertensive medications aim to inhibit or block specific metabolic processes in order to suppress reactions that drive blood pressure up. To increase effectiveness, drugs are often prescribed in combination.

Prevent that dry cough

Long-term use of ACE inhibitors in particular can sometimes lead to the development of an irritating dry cough. If you often have a slight cough but no cold, ask your doctor about switching to a sartan (angiotensin ll receptor inhibitor, see page 147).

ACE inhibitors

This group of medications includes the active ingredients captopril, enalapril, lisinopril, and ramipril as well as other chemicals ending in -pril. ACE stands for 'angiotensin converting enzyme,' a protein that converts the hormone angiotensin I into its active form, angiotensin II, which causes blood vessel contraction. If the conversion to angiotensin ll is inhibited, this effect is not triggered and the blood vessels – even those located far from the heart – remain dilated, reducing resistance to the flow of blood pumped into the circulatory system by the heart.

In addition, ACE inhibitors have been shown to protect the kidneys, making them especially useful when diabetes is also present, since long-term high blood sugar levels can cause kidney damage.

Beta blockers

This group includes active chemical ingredients such as atenolol, bisoprolol, carvedilol, metoprolol, nebivolol, and propranolol as well as other compounds with names ending in -olol. Beta blockers are among the oldest and most reliable anti-hypertensive medications. They block specific receptor sites for the hormones adrenaline and noradrenaline, which work within the sympathetic nervous system to increase heart rate and raise blood pressure. In the kidneys, beta blockers slow down production of the hormone renin, which causes blood vessels to constrict. As a result, beta blockers reduce heart rate and lower blood pressure.

Many large-scale studies have shown that beta blockers can reduce mortality, especially in cases of overly rapid heart rate (tachycardia) that are not related to lack of physical activity. Beta blockers are useful even when high blood pressure has already damaged the blood vessels, coronary heart disease is already present, and a heart attack or stroke may have occurred already. Due to undesired side effects such as impotence and perceptual disorders, however, beta blockers are not popular with patients.

Diuretics

This group includes active pharmaceuticals such as hydrochlorothiazide, furosemide, torasemide, xipamide, and spironolactone. Hydrochlorothiazide is often combined with ACE inhibitors or sartans. Furosemide und torasemide are so-called loop diuretics. They are exceptionally effective diuretics but also flush out many salts. Spironolactone is a potassium-sparing diuretic that causes the kidneys to eliminate table salt (sodium chloride) but very little potassium. Spironolactone is used primarily in cases of cardiac insufficiency because studies have shown that it effectively reduces mortality.

All diuretics drive water out of the body by causing the kidneys to pull more salt (and thus also more water) out of the tissues for elimination. For hypertension, however, diuretics must be prescribed only in very low doses to avoid eliminating too many salts (especially potassium) along with the water. Potassium deficiency in the blood can lead to cardiac arrhythmias (disturbances in heartbeat rhythm).

Calcium inhibitors

This group includes pharmaceuticals such as amlodipine, diltiazem, nifedipine, nitrendipine, verapamil, and other compounds ending in -dipine. Calcium inhibitors block the flow of calcium into the muscle cells that normally act to constrict blood vessels. If the influx of calcium is inhibited, the blood vessels remain dilated and blood pressure drops. Diltiazem and verapamil also slow heart rate, while nifedipine and other -dipines tend to speed it up, with the exception of amlodipine, nitrendipine, and delayed-release nifedipine. Studies have shown that amlodipine and nitrendipine reduce mortality from heart attacks and strokes. This is true of other calcium inhibitors only when they are administered in combination with other anti-hypertensive drugs such as ACE inhibitors or diuretics.

Timed-release medication

Hypertensive patients taking nifedipine must only receive the extended-release form of the drug, because studies have shown that otherwise it actually *increases* the risk of heart attack or stroke.

Sartans (angiotensin II receptor inhibitors)

This group includes medications such as candesartan, losartan, telmisartan, valsartan, and others with names ending in -sartan. Sartans block the effects of the hormone angiotensin II by occupying its receptor sites. As a result, the blood vessels remain dilated and blood pressure drops. Sartans are subjected to almost as much testing as ACE inhibitors and are therefore on a par with them. They also have positive effects on the heart's pumping force and are therefore suitable for use when cardiac insufficiency is already present. They can also reduce complications of high blood pressure such as heart attack, stroke, and kidney failure, especially when diabetes is also present.

Anthroposophical medicines

Anthroposophical medicines aim to counteract imbalances in a patient's constitution. In most cases, they do not produce a rapid, steep drop in blood pressure but serve as more of a long-term alterative therapy. As a rule, these medications need to be taken for two months before it is possible to tell whether they are working and how lasting the effects may be. Because they have few undesired effects, there is no reason to avoid long-term use, even for years. A time-tested practice is to administer these medications rhythmically – eight weeks on followed by four weeks off.

Some aspects of these medications may seem strange to you: why is meteoric iron supposed to be able to strengthen will forces? How does phosphorus carry light into the body, where it activates metabolism? In the descriptions that follow, we will attempt to convey at least the basic points in support of the use of these medications. Many things begin to make sense when you make the effort to observe a plant closely: its growth pattern, the arrangement of its leaves, the shape of its flower, and other details all tell us about its properties and features, often revealing therapeutic qualities. The same is true of metals and minerals.

147

Anthroposophical Medicine

Anthroposophical medicine draws on three sources: scientific medicine; a holistic understanding of the natural world; and spiritual scientific knowledge of the human soul and human existence. It is not an 'alternative' medicine in that it does not aim to replace conventional medicine. It applies all the useful knowledge that scientific research has yielded: medical technology, laboratory tests, medications, surgical procedures, and intensive care. In addition, it makes use of a variety of medicines derived from nature. Last but not least, it considers each person's personality and the unique aspects of his or her life. Treatment must be individualised, because every human being is unique.

Anthroposophical medicine makes use of some therapeutic methods that involve the patient passively (such as massages and rubs, wet packs and compresses) and others that require active participation – specifically, artistic therapies such as speech formation, music, painting, and modelling, as well as curative eurythmy, talking therapies (psychotherapy, biography work), nutrition, physical activity, physical therapy, and relaxation methods.

Pharmaceutical therapy consists in part of nature-based anthroposophical medicines, their composition determined by the typical characteristics of an illness, but also includes other remedies that are oriented towards the patient's individual constitution and designed to stimulate self-healing forces. The medicine the doctor selects (whether a full-strength extract or a homeopathic potency) depends on the nature and course of the disease, its symptoms and duration, the patient's energy level and age, and especially his or her inner and outer activity. Conventional medications are also administered as needed.

Always ask your doctor!

Never attempt to treat high blood pressure on your own. Consult your primary care physician first. If he or she does not respect your wish to lower your blood pressure through natural means, seek out a naturopathic physician, who is sure to support your efforts.

Medicine for our times

Anthroposophical medicine is truly modern because it considers each person's entire personality. Patients no longer want to be reduced to their illness. Instead, they want to be involved in their own treatment in partnership with their doctor – an important step towards individuals taking responsibility for their own health.

Cardiodoron

Cardiodoron (available by prescription only; drops and alcohol-free Cardiodoron Rh tablets) contains extracts of three plants: cowslip, henbane, and Scotch thistle. Except for Scotch thistle, which contains alkaloids that can slow an overly rapid heartbeat, the plants' connections to the cardiovascular system are not immediately apparent. Rather than being substance-based, their effects derive from the plants' essential characters. Cowslip, henbane, and Scotch thistle represent two poles and their balancing centre, and as such they stimulate the balancing forces of the rhythmic system (heart and circulation).

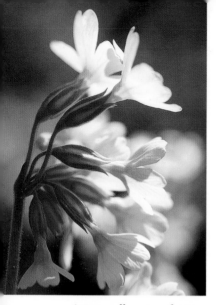

A sunny yellow sign of spring: the cowslip, formerly called 'key of heaven'.

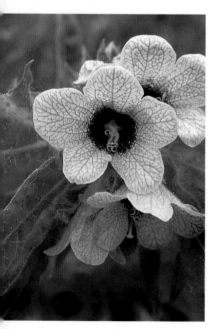

Henbane flowers are small and inconspicuous.

☞ Cowslip (*Primula veris*), with its sweet fragrance and delicate pale yellow flowers, is a typical symbol of spring. As its old name 'key of heaven' indicates, it represents the growth-enhancing force of light. Cowslip blooms immediately after the snow melts, when the soil is still very cold and damp, so its growth results less from warmth than from the force of light. It concentrates this life force and is then also able to activate it in the human body. Cowslip also contains saponins, soap-like compounds that allow water and air to mingle, producing foam. This process is related to breathing, which is closely associated with the heart's activity. Gases and fluids combine during the process of gaseous exchange in the pulmonary alveoli, where oxygen from the inhaled air is absorbed into the blood and carbon dioxide is released from the blood into the exhaled air. In the body's capillaries, oxygen is released to the tissues and carbon dioxide is absorbed into the blood. Cowslip's saponins allow it to stimulate these processes.

☞ Henbane (*Hyoscyamus niger*) has properties that make it the polar opposite of light-filled cowslip. It grows around the edges of civilized places – for example, on garbage dumps. The violet-brown veined flowers give off an unpleasant odour. Henbane represents the earthly counterpart to the 'keys of heaven' and brings their forces 'down to earth'. Its clearly structured arrangement of flowers and leaves results in a rhythmic display of seed pods along the stem. As a result, henbane has a connection to the heart as a rhythmical system. It contains the alkaloids hyoscyamine and scopolamine, which have antispasmodic effects even in small quantities, slowing an overly rapid heartbeat and lowering blood pressure.

☞ Scotch thistle (*Onopordum acanthium*) is a biennial plant. In its first year, it develops only a ground-hugging rosette of leaves above a substantial taproot. It is not uncommon for the second-year plant with its attractive candelabra-like branching pattern to achieve a height of 2.5 metres (8 ft). This growth pattern reveals the strength of Scotch thistle's vital structural forces. At the same time, forces of degeneration are also evident: the large leaves close to the ground wilt and die off early, even before the plant blooms. By late autumn, the robust taproot has completely deteriorated and the beautiful silvery, pale green top growth has been reduced to a brown skeleton that topples in the first gust of wind. As with all thistles, the large, pointed, sharp-edged prickles reveal strong formative forces and give the plant a regal and unapproachable appearance, but at the same time its graceful, expressive form and delicate purple flowers always attract attention. In Cardiodoron, only the flowers are used. They are representative of the properties of the plant as a whole but also have a close connection to the soul because they speak to the world of sensation and emotion. The flowers, because they attract insects and nectar-sipping birds, are where growth forces and

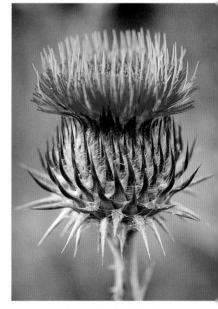

The tips of Scotch thistle's thorny branches support delicate violet blossoms.

151

soul forces meet. The plant's reproduction depends on the pollination services of these creatures, which in turn depend on the plant's nectar. Plant and pollinators exist for each other. These two qualities are also united in the heart: the bloodstream is an expression of life and as such is regulated by the forces of sensation and emotion that influence heart rate. Scotch thistle flowers, with their concentrated packages of generative and degenerative forces, strengthen both the interaction of life and soul in the body and rhythmic processes throughout the organism.

What does 'Metallicum praeperatum' mean?

'Metallicum praeperatum' (abbreviated 'met. prep.') at the end of the name of a homeopathic medicine indicates that the product is derived from a metallic mirror: the source metal (e.g., gold, silver, copper, iron) is heated in a vacuum, where it liquefies, evaporates, and then precipitates, forming a reflective surface on the inside of a glass vessel. This reflective layer is then scraped off and undergoes further processing as a powder. Through the heating process, the metal, deposited in the earth's interior millions of years ago, is purified and 'rejuvenated', restored to its pre-deposition state, namely, vapour. This corresponds to the original cosmic metal and is therefore more active and dynamic than metal, as it comes from the earth.

Aurum metallicum praeparatum (D6 to D30)

As a metal, gold has properties similar to those of the heart, which creates a rhythmical balance between the greatest possible accumulation of blood in the chambers of the heart and the blood's greatest expansion into the most distant capillaries. Gold is exceptionally dense and almost twice as heavy as lead but more malleable than any other metal. It can be rolled out into extremely fine sheets, and 1 g (less than ½ oz) of gold can be drawn out into 2 kilometres (1.2 miles) of wire. Gold supports circulatory function as a whole by strengthening and harmonising the heart's capacity for contraction and expansion.

As a medication, gold is available as Aurum metallicum praeparatum (powder, drops) in potencies from D6 to D30 (drops from D10 to D30) or in combination with plant extracts such as henbane and lavender.

Medication for stress types

In treating hypertension in stress types, it is important to make sure that their weak points are not aggravated by the side effects of conventional drugs. Other options include a number of anthroposophical constitutional remedies that can help calm over-stimulated nerves and lower blood pressure.

Conventional medication

When type-oriented treatment programmes supported by anthroposophical remedies fail to reduce blood pressure adequately, or when acute high blood pressure must be lowered quickly, ACE inhibitors or sartans are the most appropriate conventional medications for stress types. Diuretics should be used with extreme caution and in very low doses. Because stress types tend not to drink a lot of fluids, the volume of blood in circulation remains small. Diuretics would reduce it even more, and run the risk of kidney damage with long-term use.

When both blood pressure and heart rate are too high (heart rate over 90 beats per minute), a beta blocker is the prescription of choice. Stress types may seem like natural candidates for these drugs, but although beta blockers do get heart rates down to 60–70 beats per minute, they fail to resolve the underlying problem. They have never been known to help patients become more resistant or less thin-skinned, or have warmer hands or a more robust overall constitution. In fact, the slower pulse and lower blood pressure they produce tempts patients to assume everything has been taken care of and that they can just continue as before. Only very attentive individuals will notice how beta blockers suppress sensitivity as well as the problematic aspects of stress. Instead of enlivening and warming, they contribute to desensitising people to messages from the body or the soul. For this reason, it's important to do a careful assessment. Is a beta blocker really necessary, or will other antihypertensive measures suffice?

The situation is different if a heart attack has already occurred or cardiac arrhythmias such as atrial fibrillation or tachycardia (overly rapid heartbeat) are already present. In such cases, beta blockers can indeed add years to a patient's life.

Don't mix medications

Sartans *must not* be combined with ACE inhibitors. The combination increases the risk of kidney damage or kidney failure that requires dialysis, or even sudden cardiac death. These were the conclusions of a study of over 25,000 hypertensive patients treated either with the ACE inhibitor ramipril, the sartan telmisartan, or a combination of the two. These findings dashed hopes that a two-drug combination would prove more effective than either one of them alone.

Anthroposophical medicines

Anthroposophical treatments primarily target mental stress and physical depletion.

☞ Argentum metallicum praeparatum (powder, also available as drops in potencies of D8 and upward) helps to protect all vegetative processes such as blood pressure, respiration, cell division, heartbeat, digestion, body temperature, metabolism, and glandular secretion against psychologically stressful influences.

☞ Bryophyllum (propagule, powder) is a wonderful remedy for counteracting bodily depletion and restoring energy reserves. The action of the propagule extract is both calming/relaxing and restorative/strengthening. The plant's strong vegetative forces are evident in the leaf edges, where many new plantlets develop, which fall off – complete with preformed rootlets – and readily take root, hence the plant's common name 'mother-of-thousands'. Only later, when the plant has developed to full size, does it begin to flower, after which it dies, having already produced thousands of offspring. With these vegetative forces, bryophyllum primarily serves to stimulate metabolic processes, allowing you to relax and sleep better, an effect that is usually noticeable within one day.

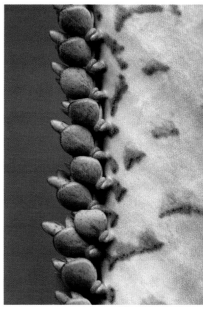

Countless tiny plants develop along the edges of the bryophyllum leaves.

☞ Hyoscyamus Rh D3/D6 (henbane, drops; prescription required for D3) is helpful when you are under great mental pressure. It contains scopolamine and hyoscyamine, which make the heart beat less rapidly and lower blood pressure. These mechanisms also mean that henbane promotes relaxation.

☞ **Aurum/Hyoscyamus comp.** (drops) is henbane (see page 150) combined with gold and antimony (Stibium). This remedy is especially valuable when blood pressure that has become derailed is associated with nervous extrasystoles (momentary arrhythmia) and anxiety.

☞ **Hyoscyamus/Valeriana** (drops, prescription required) has balancing and relaxing effects when blood pressure that rises (or fails to drop) at night makes it hard to fall asleep or stay asleep. In addition to henbane, this combination remedy contains valerian, a well-known natural sleep aid.

☞ **Aurum/Belladonna comp.** (drops) is the appropriate remedy for stress types who tend to be overweight and get red in the face when their blood pressure rises. In addition to gold and henbane, it also includes Belladonna D10, which counteracts congestion and hardening and has antispasmodic effects – just the right thing for people who tense up easily under stress.

☞ **Aurum/Lavandula comp.** (ointment) can be applied to the heart area as a compress in the evening and left on overnight. The effects are tremendously comforting and relaxing. The ointment contains gold along with lavender and rose – you'll notice the pleasant fragrance immediately.

☞ **Neurodoron** (tablets), a combination medication consisting of Aurum metallicum praeparatum, Kalium phosphoricum, and Ferrum-Quartz, is a universal anti-stress remedy. Gold has balancing, harmonising effects on circulation. Potassium (Kalium) is involved in all metabolic processes on the cellular level; phosphorus is a vehicle of light and warmth. In compound form, these two elements intensify anabolic metabolism. In addition, the combination of iron (Ferrum) with quartz and sulfur in Ferrum-Quartz creates a bridge between respiration and metabolism. The effect of the Neurodoron formula as a whole is to invigorate all metabolic processes and give new energy to a weakened body.

Homeopathic potentisation

Homeopathic medicines are always 'potentised.' This means that the starting material – usually a 'mother tincture' (a full-strength extract of a medicinal plant) – is diluted 1:10 (for D potencies), 1:100 (for C potencies), or 1:50,000 (for LM potencies) with distilled water. So 'D3' means that the original material underwent three dilutions, each in a 1:10 ratio.

My personal tip
A calming heart compress

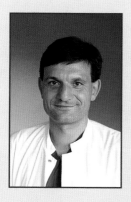

To make a heart compress, spread Aurum/ Lavandula comp. ointment about 1 cm (⅓ in) thick on a cloth handkerchief folded to about the size of the palm of your hand. Place the compress ointment-side down on your chest over your heart and leave it on overnight while you sleep. (The compress will usually stay in place if you pull a close-fitting undershirt or vest on over it.) You can re-use the compress repeatedly until it no longer smells fresh, then wash the handkerchief in a hot wash cycle. This heart compress is also a favourite with restless, fidgety children!

Medication for abdominal types

With abdominal types, the main point is to manage conventional antihypertensive therapy so that it supports rather than hinders your efforts to become active. In addition, a variety of anthroposophical medicines are also worthwhile.

Conventional medication

The most suitable conventional drugs are chemicals that intervene in kidney metabolism to prevent the release of hormones that constrict blood vessels. Drugs in this category, which includes ACE inhibitors (see page 144) and sartans (page 143), also protect the kidneys – an additional advantage and especially important if you are already diabetic or pre-diabetic. If possible, abdominal types – at least those without organ damage and who have not had a heart attack or stroke – should *not* be treated with beta blockers (see page 145). Drugs in this category tend to intensify depression and weight gain. Since beta blockers produce a sleepy, sluggish mood by inhibiting the sympathetic nervous system, it comes as no surprise that their potential to suppress independent activity and interest in the surrounding world can be counterproductive for abdominal types.

In addition to ACE inhibitors or sartans, a prescription diuretic may also make sense for abdominal types, because it prevents the body from being flooded with accumulated fluids. Diuretics are often overprescribed, however, so make sure that your doctor begins with the lowest possible dosage. Adequate daily doses are: 12.5 mg of hydrochlorithiazide or chlorthalidone, 2.5 mg of indapamide, 10 mg of xipamide, 20 mg of furosemide, 6 mg of piretanide, or 25 mg of spironolactone. These quantities should only be increased if it becomes obvious that the current dosage has failed to reduce the patient's blood pressure.

> ## Beta blockers reduce tension
> ## – and motivation!
>
> Taking a beta blocker just before a major performance can reduce a nervous person's stage fright, leaving just enough stress for effective stage presence. However, this effect is totally undesirable in abdominal types, who naturally tend to be easygoing. Beta blockers only make sense when there is a need to protect the internal organs from the constant 'whipping' of overstimulated sympathetic nerves.

Anthroposophical medicines

A number of constitutional remedies are suited to balancing out the typical one-sidedness of abdominal types:

☞ **Ferrum sidereum** (meteoric iron, D10 and D12 in powder form, D20 as tablets), is derived from meteorites that have fallen to earth from outer space. This cosmic iron is very young compared to earthly iron ores. Because an iron atom lies in the centre of each molecule of the red blood pigment hemoglobin, iron is the metal that serves respiration in the blood. Its ability to transport oxygen and carbon dioxide allow it to link respiration with metabolism. As it stimulates healthy metabolic activity, iron is also the prerequisite for a strong will. Meteoric iron is taken for two months, followed by a two month break; this rhythm can be repeated as long as necessary.

☞ **Ferrum metallicum praeparatum** (powder) is earthly iron that has been 'rejuvenated' by creating a metallic mirror (see page 152). It is formulated to support will development and the other effects of meteoric iron.

☞ **Cuprum metallicum praeparatum** (powder) is copper that is also produced by creating a metallic mirror. It has warming and anti-

159

spasmodic effects, activates metabolism, and enhances sensitivity. It is useful for lowering high blood pressure due to congestion and an overly compact body.

☞ **Hypericum auro cultum, herba** D2 and D3 (drops, by prescription only), homeopathically prepared St. John's wort, is a time-tested remedy for depression. It is manufactured from plants fertilised for three years with homeopathic dilutions of gold. This process enhances the plant's light-related qualities and makes it even more effective in brightening mood.

Medication for chaos types

For chaos type patients, 24-hour blood pressure monitoring is especially important in order to figure out *when* and *why* their blood pressure rises. When should they take steps to counteract high blood pressure, and what is the best way to proceed? Medications are selected accordingly.

Conventional drugs

Chaos types are natural candidates for ACE inhibitors or sartans. Beta blockers are not good for them at all because they constrain blood pressure in a way that allows almost no variability.

It is important for the doctor to adjust dosage very carefully and to prescribe the lowest possible dose, because chaos types' blood pressure usually stabilises on its own with appropriate alterations in their personal circumstances. Restoring natural inner balance is of primary importance and lifestyle changes have much more impact than any pill.

Anthroposophical medicines

All constitutional remedies that influence the body's rhythms are effective for chaos types:

☞   Cardiodoron (drops; see page 149).
☞   Aurum metallicum praeparatum (drops; see page 153).
☞   Aurum/Belladonna comp. (drops; see page 156).

Additional therapies

In this section, we will give brief descriptions of additional therapies used in anthroposophical medicine. They may already be familiar from the patient case histories.

Curative eurythmy

Eurythmy is an art of movement developed in the early twentieth century by Rudolf Steiner, the founder of anthroposophical spiritual science. For medical purposes, it is practised in the form of curative eurythmy, which makes use of speech, sounds, gestures, and music, transforming them into specific movements. Each sound, whether a consonant or vowel, corresponds to its own particular gesture. The underlying assumption is that there is a close connection between the movement qualities of these sounds and life processes in the body, and that this connection can be exploited for therapeutic purposes.

In consultation with the attending physician, curative eurythmists select individual sounds and gestures that they then practise intensively with the patient to achieve the desired therapeutic effects. These exercises have specific strengthening and regulating effects on rhythmic processes, especially circulation and respiration, but they also influence the activity of internal organs and general mobility and balance. Once mastered, they are easy to integrate permanently into daily routines.

Effects on organ function

Curative eurythmy has profound effects on organ function and is therefore especially appropriate in cases of high blood pressure in which not only soul and spirit but also metabolic and organic functions need to be brought into balance.

Talent not required!

Anthroposophical art therapies do not require any particular artistic talent. Rather, they are designed to aid self-discovery and help you step outside of your daily reality by finding your own spiritual dimension.

Anthroposophical art therapies

Anthroposophical art therapies (painting, sculpture, music, singing, and speech formation) help to restore the inherent harmony of body and soul.

No special ability is required; you do not need to master a musical instrument or even be musically gifted, be able to make pottery or draw well. In all art therapies, the experience is the most important thing. For example, what do I sense when I apply red and blue watercolour paints? What images rise up in me when I shape a lump of clay in a particular way? How do I feel when I pluck the strings of a harp or beat a drum?

Active involvement with clay, wood, stone, or colour; with pitches, melodies, and instruments; with speech and singing – these all allow senses that have become dulled to perceive, hear, see, and feel in different ways. As a result, you discover new and creative ways to approach your surroundings and your own inner world – including new ways to deal with illness and emotional problems.

Rhythmical massage

The art of rhythmical massage was developed in the first half of the twentieth century by two physicians, Dr Ita Wegman and Dr Margarethe Hauschka. It is based on classical massage therapy but uses different techniques and also has a different purpose. In classical massage, the muscles and connective tissues are pressed, pounded, rolled and kneaded to relax tension and stiffness. In contrast, rhythmical massage uses suction and rhythmic pulsing and stroking movements to stimulate fluid flow in the body in order to release stiffened and compacted structures. To optimise the effect, a rest period of at least 30 minutes is required after each treatment.

Rhythmical massage makes both body and soul more permeable and alert. It also lowers blood pressure by warming the body, enhancing respiration, and improving insomnia, fatigue, exhaustion, pain and congestion.

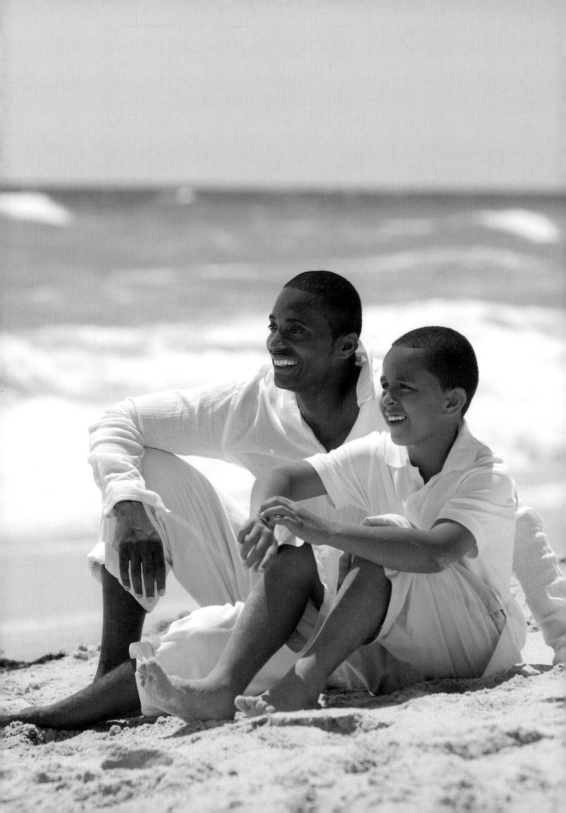

Index

The Quiet Heart
Putting Stress In Its Place

Peter Grunewald

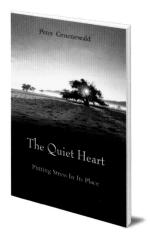

This book describes a highly effective approach to stress management and personal development. Using heart-based exercises that help manage and transform extreme emotions, it is possible to deal with many forms of stress, anxiety and depression, without resorting to drugs or psychotherapy. The benefits of these unique, easily practised exercises can be felt within days.

This updated edition contains new relaxation and self-motivation exercises, and a wider variety of case studies demonstrating real results. There is also a useful Question and Answer section which addresses common queries which have arisen since the publication of the first edition.

This book is an essential read for anyone who wants to take their physical and emotional health into their own hands.

florisbooks.co.uk

Healthy Body, Healthy Brain
Alzheimer's and Dementia Prevention and Care

Jenny Lewis

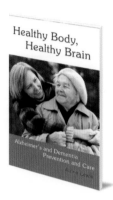

'It would benefit every household to have a copy of this book.'
– New View

This practical book is the result of Jenny Lewis's research and experience as a carer for her mother, who has suffered from senile dementia for fifteen years. In this book, she shares her advice.

Jenny speaks about the importance of valuing and caring for the elderly in our society, of encouraging mobility and independence for as long as possible. There is an emphasis on the prevention of Alzheimer's and dementia through nutrition, physical activity and maintaining a positive attitude to life, as well as suggestions on how to improve the health and well-being of those already suffering from these conditions. Jenny goes on to discuss residential care and nursing homes, and the importance of adopting a new approach towards caring for the elderly in our society.

This encouraging guide includes practical suggestions that can easily be introduced into daily routines, such as recipes for nourishing soups and brain gym exercises.

florisbooks.co.uk